Dying to Be Perfect

Dying to Be Perfect

A MOTHER'S STORY
OF HER SON'S BATTLE
WITH ANOREXIA

Susan Barry

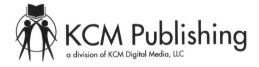
KCM Publishing
a division of KCM Digital Media, LLC

Cover design: Deena Warner Design
E-book design and production: India Amos and Peter Costanzo
Paperback design and composition: India Amos

Publisher: Michael Fabiano

ISBN 978-1-939961-00-6 (ePub Edition)
ISBN 978-1-939961-01-3 (Mobipocket Edition)
ISBN 978-1-939961-02-0 (Paperback Edition)

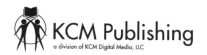

KCM Publishing
a division of KCM Digital Media, LLC

I DEDICATE THIS BOOK to my daughter, Jessica Brooke. She was okay with being put on the "back burner" while—at a very young age—she encouraged me to save her brother. She loved so much what was on the "front burner." She watched me try to save him for almost nine years. Eventually, she became frustrated and angry that nothing was working.

All the while, she was just simmering gently on the back burner. It is incredible that she turned out to be so amazing. She became beautiful and strong and independent with a huge and tender heart. She was the best sister TJ could ever have had. I am so proud of her and I could not possibly love her more.

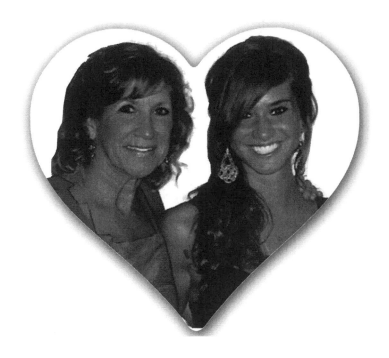

CONTENTS

FOREWORD

I was introduced to Susan Barry in early 2012 by Mary Murray, who had produced a segment on Susan and her son TJ for NBC Nightly News. She sent Susan's manuscript to me and urged me to take a brief look.

I will never forget reading the first ten pages on my train ride home from New York City. The story was astounding and I couldn't believe that Susan had summoned the courage to write in such detail and with such immense clarity about the process of losing her son to anorexia. I devoured the manuscript in a single night and I knew that I wanted the world to hear TJ's story.

Dying to Be Perfect is not intended to dispense specific medical advice or be the definitive guide on how to handle anorexia. It is meant to help readers on all sides of this pressing problem be more aware of the symptoms and challenges associated with eating disorders and how to deal with them—as a sufferer, a family member, a teacher, a colleague, or a friend. In telling one very personal story, Susan bravely shines a light on a disorder that is more widespread among both sexes and all socioeconomic groups than most people realize.

Every anorexic's story is different and personal. If you have encountered the disorder, you will recognize many aspects of TJ's story, and the way anorexia can threaten to overwhelm not just the victim but his or her entire family circle. Once you have met Susan and TJ, you won't feel alone in the struggle.

The book includes excerpts from TJ's own writings as

well as commentary by his family and friends—and one young man, TJ's best friend Daniel, who conquered the disorder—providing a multi-faceted perspective on TJ's story and anorexia in general.

The threat of losing a child is an unbearable notion to any parent. Having three children of my own, I can't imagine going through what Susan faced. The fact that she emerged from her experiences with a burning desire to help others in her situation is a testament to her own strength and passion. I share her hope that this story helps save young lives by raising awareness, inspiring action and offering advice and support to all engaged in this life-or-death struggle.

My special thanks to Susan, her family, and TJ (working his magic through us mortals) for the privilege of working on this project and helping bring it into the world.

Following are some excerpts from the many letters sent to Susan by people that read this story.

MICHAEL FABIANO
KCM Publishing—CEO and Publisher

EXCERPTS OF LETTERS
TO SUSAN*

"You have used your words so caringly and passionately and lovingly and honestly to tell TJ's story and yours too. I have been reading your book and literally can hardly put it down. It has given me such a deeper understanding of what it means to have an eating disorder, both for the patient and those who love him/her."

"TJ touched the life of everyone he met with his smile and compassion. We must use this pain as a catalyst for change."

"I feel blessed to have known such a wonderful young man. Your book is so powerful because your mother's pain is so raw. It touched my very soul."

"So much of what you said about the person TJ was and what he went through mirrors my son. My family has been at a loss for getting proper treatment and understanding how this illness has overtaken his life."

"I just finished your book. Your strength and courage amazes me. To know that you not only lived it, but then went through the whole, painful process again to put it down in words, in the hopes of maybe saving some other family the pain that all of you went through. It showed

---

* Edited with permission.

strength of spirit and courage that few people in the world have."

"What I found most interesting about TJ's story was how his drive and perfectionism fueled both his impressive accomplishments and his anorexia. My son shared those personality traits."

"I learned that if your child is anorexic, you need to take action before that 18th birthday when you will no longer have the control you are going to need to beat the disorder."

"We are just starting our battle with anorexia and the reality of what can happen is frightening. Thank you for putting TJ's story out there. I hope we are able to save our son."

ACKNOWLEDGMENTS

I WANT TO THANK the following people who have helped and encouraged me to keep going ("When is the book going to be done?!") when I was trying so hard to think of anything else. Many family and friends thought writing this book was therapeutic, but it was not. I would have much preferred playing tennis, going out to lunch, taking a walk with a friend, etc. But I knew I had to do it. The first year after TJ died, I couldn't do anything. In the second year, when I started the book, I could only write while on vacation—on a friend's balcony or by an ocean. I handwrote it and the words just flew onto the paper as though someone were helping me. But I also had help down here on earth.

Thank you to my incredible husband John, who has more patience than any human being I have ever met. His love and support are so needed and so appreciated.

Thank you to Nancy Weis, my friend since we were 5 years old. She is an avid reader and her editing and suggestions are deeply appreciated.

Thank you to Bev Wegener, my friend with whom I played on softball and volleyball teams. She spent at least 40 hours typing all those handwritten pages and did it happily . . . with breaks for hugs and tears.

Thank you to Terry Such, my friend at Such Media, who helped me with the photos, design and layout, and donated her time, expertise and creativity to my cause.

I would like to thank from the bottom of my heart, Mary Leone, whose computer expertise was absolutely invaluable to me and my publisher. She rescued me countless times when I went into panic mode.

Thank you to Mary Murray from NBC, Michael Fabiano, my publisher and Laura Ross, my editor. The blending of their collective expertise with their empathetic heart for my cause was simply unbelievable.

Finally, thank you to my son TJ. Words cannot express how much I appreciated his help. Only he knows what I mean.

Dying to Be Perfect

INTRODUCTION

IT IS TRULY a parent's worst nightmare to lose a child. It just isn't how it's supposed to be. It is almost unbearable. But, to lose a child to an eating disorder seems like a particularly senseless tragedy, because all he has to do to save himself is eat. It is so simple, such an easy and fun cure for an illness . . . at least that is how it seems to the rest of us.

My husband, John, who has been battling multiple sclerosis for more than 20 years, simply couldn't understand our son's problem. He told TJ that if he knew there was a bowl on a table 100 miles away that contained a cure for MS, he would drag his body over the cement highway to get to it. Our son's "cure" was right in our kitchen.

We watched this insidious disease overtake our "perfect" TJ during the course of nine long, painful years. I say "overtake" because I believe there came a point during the illness when, like many who suffer from eating disorders, he moved from *obsessed* to *possessed*. He was no longer TJ.

As you'll discover in reading his story, we tried everything—bribery and rewards; supporting and ignoring; tough love; umpteen therapists, dieticians and hospitals; residential treatment centers (three times); and commitment against his will for treatment (twice).

At the end, I know TJ wanted to get well. The subject line of one of his last emails to me read, "Hold me, hold me, hold me." When I opened it, I saw that he had written, simply, "Mom, why can't someone fix this?"

Most people misunderstand eating disorders, presuming that all an anorexic has to do is *decide* to eat—that he can control his eating and exercise habits; that he can refrain from throwing up if he chooses to. I'm here to tell you it is *not* that easy. As caretakers, we think that if we can find just the right words to say or prove just how detrimental these actions are to our child's health and happiness, he will just snap out of it. Sadly, this is not true either.

Another misconception is that only girls suffer from eating disorders. Many books have been written about the female struggle with body image and extreme dieting, while very little is available on the male side. (Even TJ himself felt constantly embarrassed to be grappling with a "girl's disease.") One of the reasons that I chose to tell his story was to shine a light on the many cases of male anorexia, and to offer comfort to those families who feel they are battling this version of the disease alone. But, of course, I hope that TJ's story will speak to and help families of anorexics of either gender.

I am aware of the fact that some readers might feel I am bragging about my son as I detail his many accomplishments. This is not my intent; TJ truly disliked my bragging about him to anybody for any reason. My purpose is simply to let you know TJ—what he was like and what he achieved—and in that way to help you understand that no matter how capable, talented, intelligent, informed, disciplined, or loved a child is, this illness can take hold. It is often the brightest, most motivated and promising young people who succumb to its power. An eating disorder can take over any child, from any background or situation—and it is a formidable force to reckon with.

I've found that the best way to help my friends and relatives understand this illness is to compare an anorexic to someone who is bipolar or battles schizophrenia. In all of these cases, common sense and good advice just don't constitute a cure. Even therapy can fail to make headway. All we can do is treat the illness with everything we've got and hope for a cure. Nobody chooses to be bipolar or schizophrenic—and nobody chooses to be anorexic. *It is an illness.*

After TJ's death, 22 boxes arrived at our home from his Marquette University apartment. One of them contained his lock box. Our local hardware store kindly opened it for us. We knew that our son had been consumed with making and saving money, so we expected to find his valuable coins, sports cards, stock investments, money, etc., inside. We were shocked when every card and letter ever sent to him from family or friends came spewing out of the box. So many of them conveyed the same message: "Why are you doing this, TJ? You have everything going for you!"

Also in the box were TJ's journals, some poems he had written while in treatment, photographs he took of himself (almost too disturbing to look at), and even the beginning of a book he was writing. We are certain that he left all of this for a reason—to help others.

TJ's story is both fascinating and sad but I believe it is important for me to try to tell it. I think he'd want me to. What I offer is a mother's perspective. I hope it will help other parents facing a similar circumstance, and it might even help therapists looking for new ways to understand and treat eating disorders. I believe there is value in putting this book in the hands of every coach, teacher and counselor in our schools and universities, as well as doctors, nurses, and therapists. This disease needs to be both more understood and dealt with immediately, even if it means just handing the book to a parent whose child could be suspect. It truly could help save a life. I've witnessed it over and over again in just my community. Once people are aware of and understand anorexia, they can DO something to help. Additionally, this book can be helpful to anyone dealing with a family or friend going through any kind of addiction. The characteristics of denial, frustration, control, desperation, etc., are present in all addictions. What I don't feel equipped to do is help patients. I am fairly certain that, though TJ's story might move those who suffer from this illness, it will not move them into the kitchen to make a sandwich!

Because I want to make it clear that there is always hope for families confronting anorexia and related conditions, I have included a chapter near the end written by a survivor who is now thriving. Daniel was a close friend of TJ's whom he met during one of his residential stays, and he wrote his chapter particularly for the struggling anorexic who is truly committed to recovery.

When I first suspected TJ had an eating disorder, I went to the library. I grabbed a pile of books hoping to get insight into the condition and a plan of action. Many of the books were informative on such topics as who gets it, what signs to look for, and the effects of the illness—but, few told me *what to do*! I had to go through nine years of trial and error to learn what I wished I'd known right then.

Amazingly, during the first five years after we lost our son, 25 young adults battling eating disorders were "dropped in my lap" in hopes that I might help them. They all went to residential treatment centers as a result of my meeting with their parents, explaining the illness, and insisting that they either take action or face the possibility that they'd soon be taking a very different kind of action: picking out pictures and songs for their son or daughter's funeral. Sometimes I couldn't believe what was coming out of my mouth, but they listened. These parents moved fast, and I was awestruck by the miracles.

Now I will be able to hand this book to parents and suggest that they read Chapter 18 as soon as possible. I am totally convinced this book will save lives. I only wish I'd found something like it at the onset of my son's terribly misunderstood illness.

I am also writing this for TJ's many friends, teachers, coaches, neighbors, cousins, aunts, uncles, grandparents, and fellow college and dental students. They just could not understand why TJ, with all of his intelligence and incredible discipline and drive, could allow this illness to defeat him. Perhaps this will explain it to them in a way that is both informative and enlightening.

I am a mom, not a doctor or a therapist. But I have lived this. My journey was long and difficult, filled with earnest, well-meaning, sometimes desperate steps and missteps. It is my fervent wish that telling TJ's story will mean that for some parent . . . just maybe . . . it won't be too late.

1

Beginning at the End: February 16, 2007

"THE NEXT TIME I talk to you, Mom, I'll hear the crashing of waves through your cell phone at Aunt Barbara's. I am so jealous that you and Jess get to go there. I'll call you Friday afternoon when I am done with my last final, okay? I'm bettin' you girlies will not drive all the way to Gulf Shores without stopping to spend the night!"

These were the last words I heard my son say to me.

My daughter Jessica, my sister Karen, and I were all set to go on a vacation to Alabama together—just the girls. We were planning to visit my sister Barbara and her family.

We took TJ's bet and the three of us agreed that we would drive the eighteen hours straight, just to prove to him that we could do it. It was a grueling trip. We arrived exhausted but ready to hit the beach. We three sisters were so excited that we could be together for an entire week, as were Jessie and her cousins.

After dinner, we all played a card game called euchre and had so much fun, as we always did when we got together. Then, at around 11 p.m., I suddenly became very quiet for some reason. I couldn't even smile. I felt as if something was very wrong. I tried to shake off the feeling, assuming that I was hitting a wall, just exhausted from having driven all night. But it felt more like I was having a panic attack (or what I imagined that would feel like). I got up and left the room to give TJ a quick call. I needed to hear his voice. He hadn't called me that afternoon, as he'd promised he would. He didn't answer his cell phone so I left a frantic message: "TJ, call me back right away. I have to talk to you immediately. Please do not wait until the morning. Call right now."

I rejoined the card game but we soon decided to call it a night. While we tidied up, I confessed to my sisters that I was worried about TJ. Karen suggested that I call campus security at Marquette University in Milwaukee, where he was in his first year of dental school. I immediately said, "*No way*! He'd kill me if I did that. I can just hear him now. 'Oh, great, Mom, you called campus security?! Are you kidding me? You know I had finals and that I knew you were traveling all night long!' " Neither sister said a word. They just looked at me. After a few seconds, I relented and said, "Okay, I'll call."

"Hello? My name is Susan Barry. I have a son I haven't heard from in two days, and I was wondering if you could please check on him and make sure that he is okay."

"Yes, of course, ma'am," said a calm voice on the other end of the line, "but is it unusual that you haven't heard from your son? It has only been two days. . . ."

I told the officer that it was extremely unusual for us to go even *one* day without speaking. I asked him to please call me immediately so I could sleep. He assured me he would.

Karen and I were sharing a bedroom, while Barbara and her husband, Gus, slept across the hall. Jessie and her two cousins were upstairs. We all nestled in and Karen said, "Susan, do you want me to stay up with you until they call?" I told her no, that she should just go to sleep and that I was going to shut the light off and just rest with my cell phone on my chest. The last thing I remember doing before drifting off was saying this prayer: "Dear God, please, may the next thing I hear be TJ's voice yelling at me for calling campus security."

Ring! Ring! I quickly looked at the clock. It was 12:45 a.m. I immediately started sobbing. I knew too much time had passed for everything to be fine. I was crying when I said hello.

"Mrs. Barry? This is Father Patrick from Marquette University. I am so very sorry to have to tell you this, but I am afraid that TJ has passed away . . . he looked very peaceful when we found him, Mrs. Barry. I am so very sorry."

Waking to my sobs, my sister Karen started screaming, "No! No! No!" Barb and Gus heard the commotion and came running into our bedroom. They all sat on my bed with their arms wrapped around me. I was shaking uncontrollably while trying to write down the number I was told to call in the morning.

I really don't know how long we all sat there crying. It could have been ten minutes or two hours. We were all numb. They gently asked questions. "Do you want us to wake Jessie up? Do you want us to make any calls?" I said no to all of them, and said I would do whatever was necessary in the morning. I don't remember anything more about that night.

At some point, the night ended and morning began. I needed to call TJ's dad, but he couldn't understand what I was saying as I was crying too hard. Barbara had to take over for me.

Next, I called John, TJ's stepdad. I knew that was going to be tough, too. Poor John was in the hospital himself, battling an infection caused by complications of his MS. (I hadn't even wanted to leave him to take the vacation with the girls—but he had insisted that we have our get-away.) John had been through a lot the past few months, with TJ's condition and his own health problems. Now I had to tell him the worst news any parent can hear. We stayed on the phone for just a few minutes—what could we say to comfort each other? I promised to call him back when I had calmed down a little.

Then came my hardest chore of the morning: telling TJ's sister, who was sound asleep upstairs, still believing she had a brother. She was 16, a junior in high school. I asked Barb to please get her girls up and tell them what had happened, and let Jess be the only one left in the bedroom. When Jessie was alone, I went in, shut the door, and crawled in bed with her. I lay there awhile, just looking at her face, trying to figure out how I was going to tell her. Finally, I gently shook her awake and said softly, "Honey, TJ passed away last night."

My tears started flowing again. She searched my face, desperately trying to catch me playing a very bad joke on her.

"He did not."

"Yes, honey. He did," I choked, trying to hold back my own sobs.

"No! He didn't!" she shouted in one last attempt at denying the worst. Then she burst out crying and we hugged each other. We lay there for a long time. When I finally left the room so Jessie could be alone with her thoughts for a little while, the rest of the girls were gathered around. No one said a thing. We all reached for one another in an embracing hug.

I had to call that number I'd been given by Father Patrick at Marquette: the coroner's office. When I got through, I told the lady who answered that I wanted to know about everything they'd found.

"We are very concerned about his weight," she began. "Was he on drugs?"

"No ma'am," I said. "He's never even had a beer." I paused. "He had an eating disorder."

"How old was he?"

By that time, he looked about 12. "He is 22," I told her.

"Where was his body?"

"He was on the floor."

I told her he was probably doing sit ups and she agreed. "He was on a mat. There were two space heaters on and the room was 88 degrees. Was that to sweat more?"

"No," I sighed. "It was to keep warm. He had zero body fat."

"He had a full plate of food ready to eat in the kitchen," she added, and of course I could picture it vividly.

She gave me a few seconds with my thoughts and then went on to tell me that they were required by law to do an autopsy. I felt as if I was going to pass out. I thanked her, hung up, and sat on the bed, unable to stop sobbing and trembling uncontrollably, as if an unbearable chill had seeped permanently into my bones. Perhaps this was the kind of cold that TJ felt, I thought.

What the coroner didn't realize was that I could have told her every detail of what happened that night. I knew he died exercising. I knew what time his heart finally gave out. He always did his second set of 1000 sit ups from 6 to 8 p.m., and then, having completed his four daily hours of exercise (two before class and two after) as well as his homework, he would finally feel worthy of his one meal of the day. He would eat from 8 to 10 p.m. while reading and answering his email, looking at Facebook, and watching "SportsCenter."

When TJ's soul left this earth he was almost finished with his sit-ups, his food ready . . . it was probably 7:45 p.m. And of course I could have told the coroner what he'd prepared for himself: a full plate of food with zero fat, zero sugar and zero calories.

We all left the next morning to head back to Michigan. Those same long 18 hours in the car felt like three. I insisted on driving. My sisters kept trying to take over but I wouldn't let them. Two hours went by, then four, then six, then eight. . . . I only stopped when Karen suggested I might want to start writing TJ's obituary.

I could not believe I had to write an obituary for my son, and that started me crying all over again. No parent should ever have to do that. I just could not seem to pull it together. While driving, I had been in a kind of trance—but now the reality hit me hard. I had to plan my child's funeral. Lots of questions came bounding into my head at the same time. How does his body get back to Michigan? Do his dental school friends know yet? What about his apartment? When should the funeral take place? What songs should be played? What cemetery should we choose? What should he wear?

My mind was reeling. All of his clothes are at school in Milwaukee. . . . But underneath all of these technicalities, I just kept thinking, "I want to die. I need to die. I have to die. I don't want to do any of this. Why couldn't someone help my son? We tried everything possible, didn't we? Why couldn't he have had any other illness but an eating disorder? *Anything* but an eating disorder."

2

No Worries:
22 Years Earlier

I COULDN'T SLEEP. I was uncomfortable. I was nine
months pregnant with our first child. I didn't want to
wake up my husband so I got up and tried the couch,
but that didn't feel any better. I went into the bathroom
and sat on the toilet, and surprisingly, felt better in that
position. All of a sudden, I started to push . . . hard. That
felt really good!

I felt an irresistible urge to push again, even harder this
time, and I wondered why I was pushing when I hadn't
had a contraction yet. After a few more very hard pushes,
I yelled for my husband Tom.

He came bounding into the bathroom asking, "What's
wrong?"

"I haven't had any contractions but I want to *push!*" I
told him.

"Don't push!" he commanded in a firm voice.

I lumbered to my feet at his insistence but when he
saw his firstborn son's head crowning on my backside,
he turned chalk white and crumpled to the floor. "We
need to get to the hospital right away," he said shakily,
"but you're going to have to wait a second until I can get
up!"

Going 90 miles per hour to the hospital, he kept repeating, "Don't push! Sing a song!" The only song I could

think of was "Happy Birthday to You," which I sang as fast as I could.

I never made it to the delivery floor. My doctor wasn't on duty that night but my son wasn't planning to wait. So, with people milling around the emergency room and my pale husband again on the floor and asking for water, TJ was born. He came into the world without my experiencing a single contraction or one moment of pain. You could call it the perfect delivery. We named him Thomas Lee Warschefsky II and nicknamed him "TJ" after a very special student of mine.

TJ was such an easy baby. I remember people being amazed that I never had to put a bib on him, because he never spit anything out. He loved to eat.

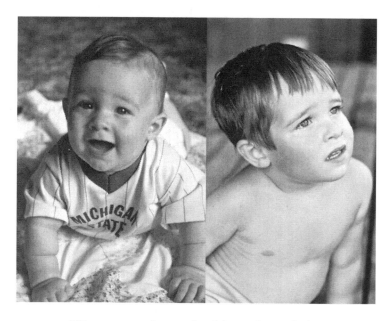

TJ was a very happy, healthy and easy baby.

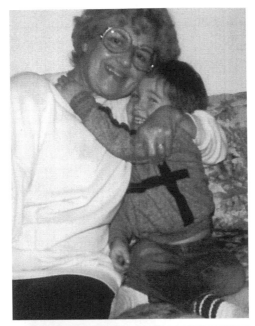

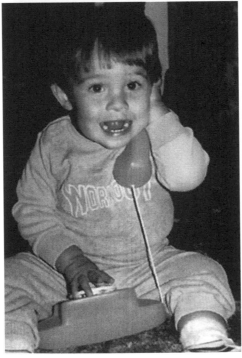

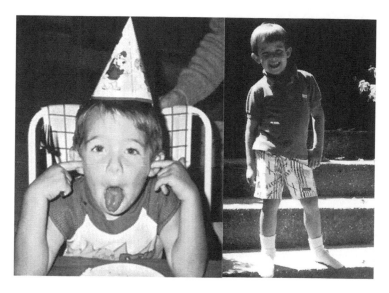

As a toddler, TJ was fun and comical and continued to be wonderful and self-sufficient. When he was 3, he would crawl out of his bed, go get a bowl of Cheerios, and turn on cartoons very quietly so he wouldn't wake me. He knew Saturday was my only day to sleep in.

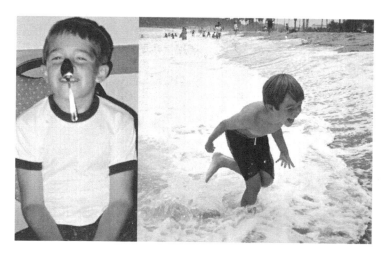

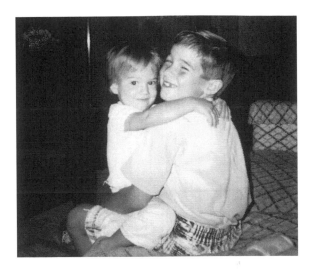

TJ and his sister were best friends.

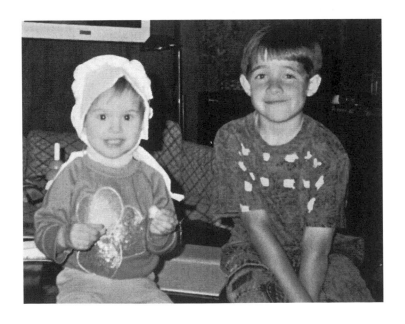

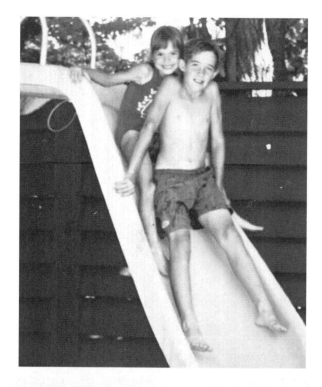

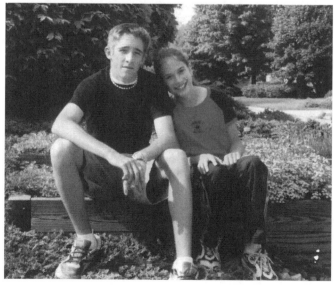

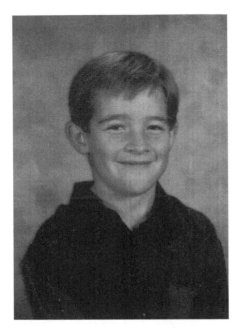

When he was about to turn 8 years old, I told TJ that he could invite eight of his closest friends and cousins to a birthday party. He got very quiet and a sad look passed over his face.

"What about the rest of the kids in my class, Mom?"

"Well . . . we don't really have room to invite everyone," I explained.

He thought for a second and said, "That's OK, Mom. I don't want a party."

Even at an early age, he was sensitive and often put the feelings of others before his own needs and desires.

His elementary and middle school years were filled with team sports at which TJ worked hard and excelled— he was more concerned with doing well on the field than in the classroom. TJ was a winner: He played just about everything and did well at anything he tried. By the time he was 4 years old he knew how to play euchre and chess,

and he could easily beat the adults at memory games. He
was always happy and had lots of friends.

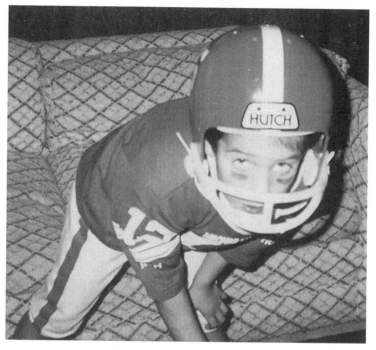

TJ played and excelled at almost every sport.

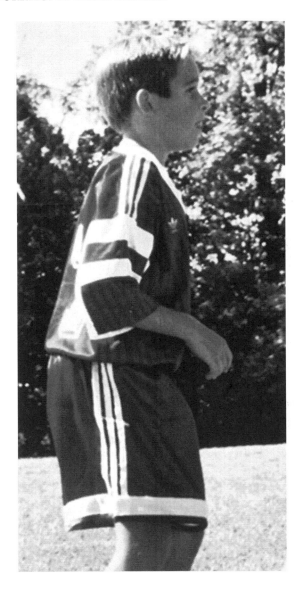

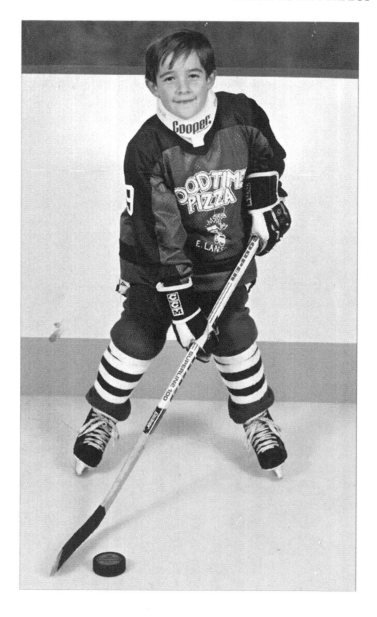

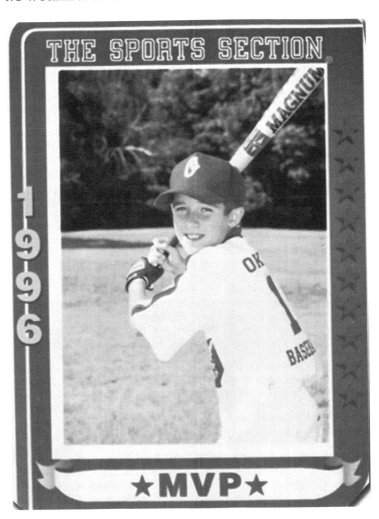

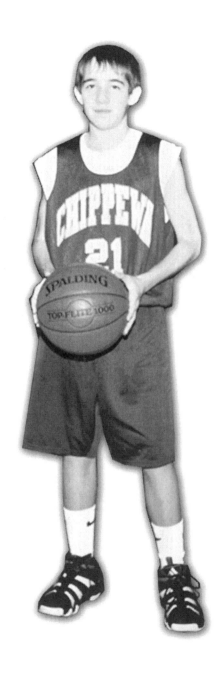

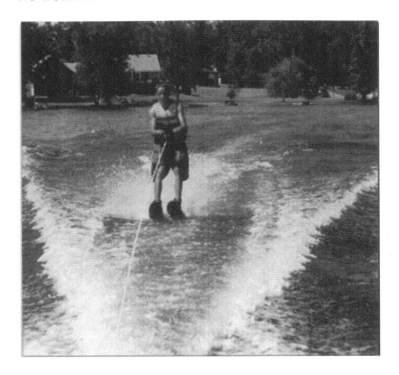

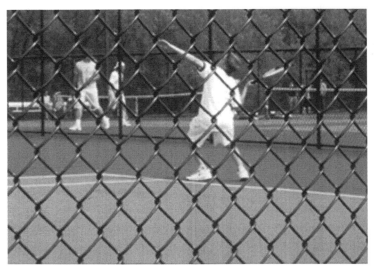

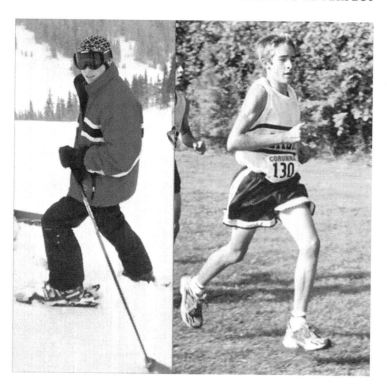

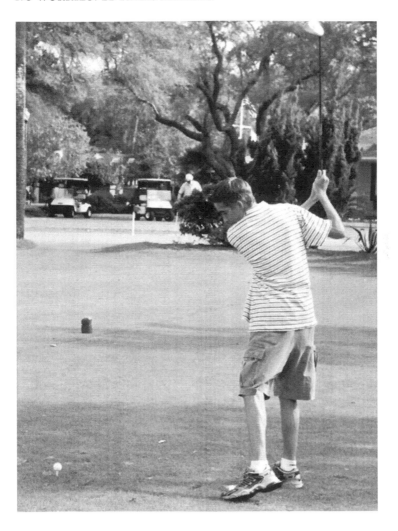

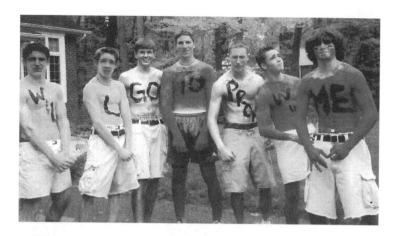

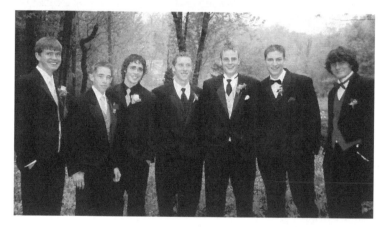

By high school, TJ's desire to excel academically kicked in ("because now it counts, Mom") and he signed up for all of the most challenging classes. He even took "Zero Hour," which added an additional class to his schedule. He was on the tennis and cross-country teams, went to all the dances, took ski and camping trips with his buddies, and continued to widen his circle of friends.

You might think I am exaggerating, but I have no reason to be anything but honest: The truth is, TJ was neat, organized, disciplined, motivated, and a straight-A student. He didn't drink, swear, have sex, or indulge in any of the vices I was prepared to deal with when he became a teenager. He didn't even laze around watching endless TV—just a few favorite things, including football and basketball games, "SportsCenter" and *Everybody Loves Raymond.*

One night, all of TJ's friends met at a local restaurant after a game and they decided to tease him a little. Knowing how much he loved to make and save money, they all started putting dollar bills in the center of the table. One buddy said, "TJ, all that money is yours. All you have to do is say *one* swear word." When he told me about it later, he said, "I didn't get the money, Mom. I'm not going to compromise my values." I told this story to one of my tennis friends and he reached into his wallet and pulled out a 20. He said, "Give this to my man TJ and tell him how proud I am of him."

Another day, when I got home from teaching, TJ was away at a tennis match. Passing by his bedroom, I saw that he'd already laid out his clothes for the next day. Next to them were his wallet, his keys and a stick of gum. Walking into his bathroom, I found that he'd put toothpaste on his toothbrush. It was 4:30 in the afternoon.

At the time, I thought that all of TJ's traits were amazing and commendable. Who wouldn't want a child like this? He worked constantly, cutting eight of our neighbors' lawns every weekend. He studied hard and got straight As. He was neat, clean, organized, and a good money-saver He was the most disciplined and motivated kid anyone knew.

In retrospect, of course, I realize that all of these stellar qualities had a dark side. They were the first signs of his compulsive perfectionism. Clearly, TJ never felt good enough and was always striving to be better. His obsessions and rituals, his rigidity about schedules and time, his black-and-white sense of morality—all of these things prefigured his looming illness.

The traits that took him far in school and sports eventually contributed to his anorexia—or were symptoms of it, I'm not sure which. He outsmarted his friends, teachers and coaches. Not one of them ever called us during his nine-year battle. Not one ever mentioned that he didn't look good, his performance was suffering, that his energy level was low, that he was cold all of the time, pale or looked like a skeleton. Not one.

Through his high school years, while we watched his weight drop dangerously and his behavior become extreme, we hoped he would spontaneously get better. That he would *choose* to get better. After all, he was TJ. He could do anything. We thought that when his condition started affecting his ability to do what he wanted to do, he could and would fix it.

Over those years, we sent him to therapists, dieticians and even a personal trainer who we hoped would convince TJ that there were ways to put on muscle without getting fat. With the help of these professionals, he did hold his own throughout high school. The therapist diagnosed him with a "fat phobia."

Everything changed on April 18, 2002, when TJ turned 18. At that point, he was officially an adult, empowered to make his own choices.

These excerpts from TJ's June 2002 application to the Honor's Institute at Albion College show how gifted he was at presenting himself. (All of the emphasis are Susan's.) What institution wouldn't be eager to take him on based on this?

For as long as I can remember, family and friends have told me how successful I would grow up to be because of my foresight and determination. I have always been a very goal-oriented individual with <u>extremely high standards for myself</u>.

I have always loved being the leader in school, athletics, and among friends, and have excelled when put in that position. It intrigues me to <u>have control</u> over what needs to be done, so it is sure to be done correctly.

Throughout high school I have maintained over a 3.9 GPA at a very competitive high school, while being involved in numerous extra curricular activities and organizations. Schoolwork has always been the first priority to me, simply because I feel that a good education is the basis for a good future. It is common for students such as myself, who enjoy athletics, community activities, and social life, to become easily distracted by these outside factors. On the other hand, I enjoy the schooling aspect of my life just as much as any other and openly accept any challenge that may lie before me in the classroom or anywhere else. Trying to fit cross-county practice, Spanish club, lifting weights, volunteer work, homework, tennis, and family all into one day (starting at 2:40 p.m.) is not very easy. Yet, this is a typical school night for me, and I feel that one of the most important aspects of my life is <u>balance</u>. I have learned the need to prioritize all of my activities and interests in order to be the most productive individual possible. Morrie Schwartz, most recognizable from the novel, <u>Tuesdays with Morrie</u>, once stated, 'Devote yourself to loving others, devote yourself to your community around you, and devote yourself to creating something that gives you purpose and meaning'. I love this quote and take ft to heart, as I attempt to model these beliefs throughout my rigorous daily schedule. I take pride in my church and religion, and participate in church events as often as possible. Finally, I try to be helpful to my elderly neighbors as I mow their lawns, shovel their snow, take out their garbage, and pick weeds for them.

For my efforts in the classroom, on the athletic field, and in the community, I have received many awards. Out of over 10,000 applicants, I won the Discover Card Tribute Award Scholarship ($2,500) for the State of Michigan, and was a finalist on the national level. I received the MEAP scholarship award. In tennis, I have earned First Team All-League Honors, as well as Academic All-League in tennis and cross-country. I was a finalist for the MHSAA Scholar Athlete of the Year award. I received the Presidential Fitness Award. I was one of 150 juniors and seniors chosen throughout the state to attend a leadership camp called the Michigan Freedom Academy 1am a recipient of the Okemos High School Student Award, and also a member of the National Honor Society I won the Kevin Miller Tribute Award Scholarship ($1000), as well as the Ann Lohman Good Sportsmanship Award ($200). These honors show what I am capable of doing, although I wish to make more of an impact through my college studies.

I started skiing when I was two years old, and since then I have picked up and competitively played over fifteen different sports. Throughout my athletic career I have been the starting goalie for my hockey teams, pitcher for my baseball teams, point guard for my basketball teams, and running back for my football teams. All of these positions are considered the "leadership positions" for their respective sports, and further goes to prove my ability to thrive as a leader (Don't these positions help control the game?) In addition to participating on these organized teams for the school and on travel teams, I lift weights for two hours every other day, play in a basketball league, play soccer, golf, as well as hunting and fishing on a recreational level. I feel that my diversity on the playing field will carry over to my business career

There have been many obstacles that I have overcome throughout my life. When I was four my parents were divorced. I felt torn between the two people I love most I learned that life is not always a paved road, and that I must not dwell on the negatives that are set before me. My mother was remarried to my stepfather who has multiple sclerosis. He cannot walk and I must help my mother with all the household chores and man-related jobs that he is unable to perform. I have a very strong desire to accomplish my goals and am extremely motivated and disciplined. I choose classes, athletics, workloads, schedules, and even friends that will help me attain these goals.

Another barrier I have fought through is my height I am short for my age, but I have made up for that with quickness, skill, and a positive attitude. Most people I know that are not very tall have given up on their sport for that reason. I lift weights and my strength makes up for this absence of height I have always believed that it was more of a mental barrier, and I have overcome this in many ways. Throughout my life I have had to stay focused through many trying times and through these hard times I have relied on my faith. Like these hardships, I will conquer any hurdle that may lie in my path during my education and athletics at Albion College.

I have a reputation of having integrity high morals, and a strong sense of right and wrong. I am not the average

Christian who goes to church on Sunday and then leaves
feeling relieved that they did their deed for the week. I
try to live each and every moment of my life as though
God was standing right next to me. This discipline to act
in a way in which I believe is correct will be an asset to
me when I get to the business world where my honesty
willpower and determination are put to the test

I believe that honesty is one of, if not the most important, characteristic a person can have. I am proud to be
trustworthy Not only is it honorable to possess honesty
and integrity but it gives me a good feeling when others
say 'Ask TJ, he doesn't lie."

I am not attracted to easy routes. I do anything that
will challenge me. As a senior, 1am taking Advanced
Placement Government, Advanced Placement Spanish,
and Honor's Physics. I have taken an extra class for three
years of high school and started an hour earlier than my
classmates. This year I lettered and excelled in three varsity sports. I have never smoked, drank or performed any
other such actions to harm my body and am extremely
disciplined, organized, and driven to go above and beyond what is expected. I do not swear, steal, lie or cheat,
nor do I involve myself with those who do. For these
reasons, I feel that I am equipped with all of the necessary
traits to make the Honor's Institute proud.

At the time, we saw no red flags in TJ's exemplary behavior. He was a motivated, self-sufficient striver who set
high goals and met them. Of course, with the benefit of
hindsight, it is easy to see all of the danger signs.

I want to end this chapter with a couple of sample
report cards and a letter of recommendation he received

in high school, all of which show his propensity to overachieve.

Okemos High School
Sixth Hour class
Name: Warschefsky, TJ   Date: Mon. Nov. 23, 1998
1) Hw chapter 18 review: 20/20
2) Test Systems Project: 40/40
3) Hw Digestive System Stories: 25/20
4) Test Nutrition: 85/87
5) Test extra credit   4/0
Weighted Average: 103.8%
Grade: A

Okemos High School
History 4th Hour
Name: Warschefsky, TJ Date: Sun. Dec. 19, 1999
1) Subtotal: 380/368
2) Test Chapter 2:   17/19
3) Homework Chapter 12:   25/25
4) Current events: 16/8
5) Homework 13.4   5/5
6) Test Chapter 3:   24/25
7) Homework Chapter 13:   31/30
8) Current events: 16/8
9) War and Peace: 20/10
10) World War I Report: 10/10
11) Test Chapter 14:   27/29
12) "Sweepstakes":   35/30
13) Homework Chapter 14:   20/20
Total Possible Points: 626/587 = 106.6%
Grade: A

To Whom It May Concern:

I am pleased to give my highest recommendation and support to TJ Warschefsky, a young man about to graduate with honors from Okemos High School. I know him well, as his teacher of both Algebra I and Algebra 2, and as his cross-country coach. TJ was an excellent math student, earning all A's and doing an outstanding job in both algebra classes. In cross country I am impressed with his athletic talent and his leadership skills.

In the classroom, TJ has had outstanding success. His ever-present sense of humor yet serious attitude toward his work has brought the respect of his teachers and peers. TJ is motivated in the academic setting, and his responsible attitude helps him shine above the others. His success in his first three years of high school has earned a placement in three advanced placement classes in this, his senior year, and induction into the honor society as well. TJ has been involved in numerous sports, school organizations, in his church and in the community He has done a great deal of community service, served as a middle school camp counselor and held down jobs to earn spending money and help save for college. TJ is motivated in all these areas and, indicative of his drive, has also taken an extra hour of school (a zero hour offered at 7AM) each term in order to take more high school courses.

TJ is a fine athlete. His performance in varsity tennis and skiing have made a great contribution at Okemos High School. I can observe in one season of running that TJ is working his way up and turning into one of our elite runners. He is physically fit, ready for a challenge, and very motivated—in the classroom, on the tennis courts, on the slopes, and generally in all he pursues. Teachers and coaches are aware of TJ's sincerity and commitment to his pursuits and admire him for this.

I would like to say something about another important characteristic that separates an exceptional young person from his peers: character TJ has the highest morals, values and respect for himself and others. I have observed this in TJ throughout his high school career, and it is a shining quality TJ enjoys his friends and fun, but always displays good, clean, and respectful behavior He has a great group of friends, and ability to live his own conscience, and he has made good decisions in his young life.

TJ, most importantly will make a great officer. As a teacher and coach for 32 years, I have known and observed many young people. In TJ, I see one of the best leaders, and one of the finest kids. TJ can take orders and give them he can be sincere and he can be fun, he can be extremely motivated and he can be 'laid back', but in all he does he demonstrates the highest of values and is a role model for his generation.

Sincerely

JQ

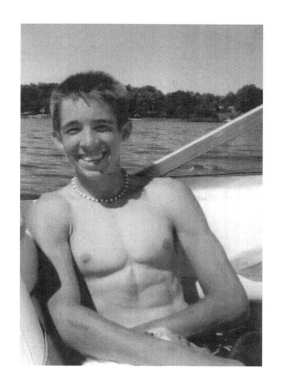

Holding Steady

3

Early Concerns

AT THE ONSET of TJ's illness, we really didn't have a clue that anything was wrong. Maybe we questioned why he was blotting his pizza with a napkin but his reply was hard to argue with: "All that grease is nasty." No big deal. His appearance didn't seem to change because his baggy clothes hid his weight loss. His multiple layers of clothing were right in style. TJ had always loved all sports, so being a very active eighth grader seemed pretty darn normal—until the soccer party.

He was on the ninth grade Okemos High School soccer team and volunteered our home for a beginning-of-the-season pool party and barbeque. I couldn't have been happier seeing him surrounded by his teammates and coaches, enjoying our backyard. It didn't take long for the boys to start taking their T-shirts off and diving into the pool. They were having a blast, cannonballing, catching footballs in midair while leaping off the diving board, and engaging in typically high-spirited teenage horseplay. John and I were sitting at the kitchen table and watching them out the window, laughing and loving the scene.

Then TJ took his shirt off. We were shocked at how thin he had become! "Oh, my gosh!" I said to John. "Look at TJ! I can see his ribs!"

After the party, I asked TJ, point blank: "How much weight have you lost? You don't look healthy, honey."

"Mom, we've been doing two-a-days in soccer practice this month," he said, brushing off my concern.

That didn't ease my mind completely. "TJ, I'm going to make you an appointment for a physical. I want to make sure there isn't something causing you to lose weight—like a tapeworm, or something." Honestly, I thought that was a possibility!

I went ahead and made an appointment with our family doctor, while TJ continued on with school and soccer as usual.

Three days after the doctor had examined him, the phone rang. It was Dr. S. and she was very agitated. "Mrs. Barry! I need TJ off the soccer team *now*! I think he has an eating disorder! His testosterone level should be at least in the 300s and it is at eight! I don't want him doing anything physical! I hardly want him walking!"

My head was spinning. "What? Wait a second! What are you talking about? What do you mean?"

Dr. S. went on to explain that she herself struggled with an eating disorder and still needed support every other weekend. She was well aware of the signs and offered to refer me to her friend, a therapist who specialized in eating disorders.

This is where denial comes into play. I thought that because she had this problem, she must be overreacting. She knew TJ cut eight lawns in the neighborhood and told me she didn't want him doing that. She said she would talk to her friend, the specialist, and get back with me.

I couldn't believe what I was hearing. I went upstairs to TJ's room. When I saw his soccer shoes on the floor, I burst out crying. How could this be happening?

The following day I told TJ what the doctor had said, and that she didn't want him playing sports or cutting lawns. He cried. I cried.

"Mom . . . Mom! I don't want to lose those lawn accounts! They're depending on me! And I've been playing soccer since I was 4 and I finally made the high school team! How can you do this to me?"

Then he went into the bargaining mode that became all too familiar as the disease progressed. He promised he would eat and gain weight if I would only give him a chance.

It broke my heart to watch his heart break. But I couldn't just forget about what the doctor had said—and the urgency in her voice.

The next day, I did two things. I talked to the soccer coach, explaining what was going on and insisting that I would have to pull TJ from the team. I asked him if he could protect TJ from embarrassment by telling his teammates that he had an injured knee. He seemed to understand and said of course he would. Then I looked in the phone book for a therapist. I didn't want to wait for the doctor to talk to her friend. I wanted to get started immediately. Of all the therapists listed in the book, only one said, "Also specializing in eating disorders." I called the number and made an appointment.

Although he wasn't happy about it, TJ allowed me to take him to the appointment. We agreed that I would pick him up in an hour. When I returned in 45 minutes, he was sitting on the curb in front of the building.

"TJ! What is going on? Why are you done so early?" I asked.

"She wants to talk to you, Mom."

I parked the car and hurried in, hoping that with the therapist's help, TJ would soon be getting better. I was shocked at what she told me.

"I'm sorry, Mrs. Barry, but I'm afraid you are going to have to take TJ to someone else. He won't talk to me at

all. I explained to him that communication can only occur when one person talks and the other responds—but
he won't talk."

I was stunned. That was it? In a shaky voice, I replied,
"Doctor, I'm a teacher. I could never tell any parent that
I'd given up on her child 45 minutes after meeting him!"

"I'm sorry," she replied, shaking her head.

That was the beginning of a nine-year nightmare.

Thankfully, TJ's doctor soon came through with the name
of an eating disorder specialist who worked at Michigan
State University. Although his practice was generally
confined to MSU athletes, he agreed to take on TJ. We
continued to see Dr. R. for the four years TJ was in high
school, and at his instruction, we also consulted a dietician. I was told to weigh TJ weekly and call his weight
in to Dr. R.

TJ was 5-foot-5 at the time. Dr. R's rule was that if he
did not weigh 110 pounds at his weekly weigh-in, we
were to prohibit him from playing on the tennis team or
running cross-country. That seemed like a good plan—a
way to rein in TJ's problem. The reality was somewhat
different.

For four straight years, every Monday morning, TJ
weighed in at exactly 110. He knew precisely what he
needed to eat and drink before each weigh-in to keep
the number on the scale where it needed to be—but
not an ounce higher. What I had thought was the best
thing to do for TJ during those four years turned out to
have the opposite effect: It only made him more adept
at hiding his problem. Because he became an expert at

micromanaging that number on the scale, he only slipped once in four years.

Starting in 2003, during one of TJ's stays at a residential treatment center, he kept a journal in which he expressed his feelings. It was one of the things we found after we'd lost him. In some of the entries, TJ looked back and described how he'd felt during the earlier stages of his illness. In this entry, he talks about the one and only time he did not make weight.

I'll never forget the day he describes here—his birthday. He knew we would all go out to eat and then have a custom-designed Baskin-Robbins ice cream cake—our family tradition. He didn't eat all day, of course, knowing he was going to have to eat a lot that night.

The year 2000 was my SWEET 16th birthday. I was supposed to be weighed the morning of my birthday but convinced my mom to let me do it the following day because I didn't want to have to deal with it on my birthday. Little did I realize that it would give me even more worries. I didn't eat all day because we were going out for a birthday dinner and dessert. I had to eat a lot to show my parents that I was okay (who was I fooling?). On the same token, I had a big varsity tennis match the following day which I could not play in unless I made weight that morning. After the dinner I stepped on the scale to see if I was going to make it. I was way far away after skipping two meals earlier in the day. From 8:30 p.m. until 10:00 p.m. that night I had an entire box of cereal, two apples, multiple glasses of juice, and over half of my birthday cake. This was all eaten immediately following a huge restaurant dinner. I literally crawled up the stairs. Hunched over and brushing my teeth is when it all came up. I went to spit out the toothpaste and everything I had eaten that night came out. By no means had I purged or done it on purpose (I never did that), but I was so stuffed that it was forced out of me. I yelled for my mom and we both spent an hour on the cold bathroom floor that night bawling our eyes out. Neither of us had the answer for this awful disease. Did anybody?

The day our son turned 18, he walked out of Dr. R.'s office forever. It was his right to do so as an adult. From that point on, I couldn't even access his medical records without his permission—in spite of the fact that I was still paying his doctor bills! That's just the way it is, I was told. Nothing we can do about it. All that followed was the sad consequence.

Ironically (and tragically), the illness TJ was fighting only picks up speed and strength after the age of 18, just as parents and other authority figures are losing their ability to help. The anorexia sufferer doesn't want help. Under its influence, the most honest kid turns into the best liar and hider on the planet. What's more, he attempts to enlist his family to help keep the disease hidden because it embarrasses him. As you can imagine, the family unit can be turned inside out by this. From what I understand, it is very much like having an alcoholic in the family. In the early stages, you enable, beg, bribe and try to get your child to listen to reason. Ultimately, you become immersed in the illness and end up colluding with him to keep it a secret.

Another journal entry reveals TJ's own perspective on his developing problem.

I got weighed almost every single week for nearly four years in order for me to play sports and do everything I wanted to do. Although after only the first month or so, I got myself into a pickle that would be a burden for each weigh-in to follow. It was weigh-in day and I knew I had no chance of making the weight. The day before I was to be weighed, I completely stuffed my mouth with anything that would fit inside of it. Sure enough, the next morning, I not only made the weight, but exceeded it by a couple of pounds. I had even gotten up early to drink numerous large glasses of water. This was great! I beat the system! I could play any sport or do whatever I wanted until at least the next weigh-in. That is just what I did. I felt free and like a normal teenage boy all week being able to play lift, run, and do whatever all week long. There was only one problem; I was not eating nearly enough to sustain my level of activity for that week. On top of that, the weight shown by the scale last week was a total spoof. There was at least two pounds of sheer water weight, and all that food in my stomach had quickly evacuated out the other end because I couldn't digest it all at one time. In fact, I weighed myself a few hours after my mom did it on that morning, and I was already four pounds lighter—and that was just after going to the bathroom a couple times! So when the next weigh-in came, I was left with no option but to load up on pounds of food and water to make it look like my weight was headed in the right direction.

This awful process followed me around throughout

high school. Just because of one week that I "had" to exercise, I was forced to completely stuff myself the day before every weigh-in for the next four years. Even if I had gained "real" weight during the previous week I would still have to stuff myself to show any progress, because I had stuffed myself the week before. I absolutely dreaded the day before a weigh-in. My mood for the entire day was horrid because I knew that I was going to have to stumble up the stairs to my bed that night and lie there for hours on end with a terrible stomachache. I would lie in bed listening to my stomach make noises that were a clear cry for mercy: "Why can't you just treat me normal every day of the week instead of starving me for six days and stuffing me for a few hours of one day?" I would stare at my ceiling, praying that I would just fall asleep so that my stomachache would just go away. However, I had to pee so much from all the water I had taken in that it was impossible to relax. If I peed, then I would lose all my water weight, so I had to hold it in all night long. I could count the hours of sleep I got on each of those nights on one hand (with a couple of missing fingers).

That was one of the most profound problems. I would only eat all that food and put on the weight because there were conditions and I was forced to. Rarely did I do it for myself, no matter what went on in my head. That is why I would have to stuff food in my gullet the night before a weigh-in; because I would not eat very much during the rest of the week because I did not have to. It was a vicious cycle that was very difficult to overcome.

Throughout high school I met with my psychiatrist every other week. I absolutely hated the man and disrespected most of the things that he said. In my mind, he was just there to make my life miserable. He would weigh me each time I went there. For a long time, I would also have to be weighed at home by my mom. I absolutely hate any scale now because of the terrible memories, if I didn't make the weight I was supposed to be at, then there were consequences that prohibited my activity. They would not let me go to the club to play basketball with my friends, I couldn't lift weights, I could not run, I could not play tennis, no sit-ups . . . nothing. That is when the lying and deceiving came forth. I absolutely love all sports for the sake of playing them (not losing weight). My friends and I were constantly active playing sports or just running around. When I was not allowed to play sports or be active, it absolutely killed me (although not eating was also killing me).

It is so shameful for a male to have an eating disorder Not one of my friends had a clue during the entire time it was going on. My parents and my psychiatrist told my coaches about the situation, and said that there might be times when I am unable to play because of my weight, but make up an injury so my friends didn't find out. During my sophomore year on JV soccer I was out five weeks with a "serious knee injury." A quick diagnostic translation on that bum knee was simply that I had lost weight and was not allowed to play until I got to a certain number. Although however much I hated eating because I was forced to and being controlled like that, I loved sports and activity so much that I would gain the weight just so I was able to play them. It was a "quick fix" more than anything. I would only do it because that was what I "had" to do in order to get what I wanted. It did not change anything in my mind because I didn't want it to.

I truly believe that having a child with an eating disorder is one of the most challenging ordeals any family can go through. If my son had cancer, for example, everyone would have understood what it was; everyone would have empathized; everyone would have wanted to help. There would have been medications, treatments, surgeries and—one hopes—a cure, or at least some answers. But when confronted with an eating disorder, people say things like:

"Why don't you just make him sit there until he eats?"

"Send him to our house. I'm a good cook."

"Does he just want to be the center of attention?"

"Maybe he loves controlling the whole household."

"He must have a low self-esteem."

"Why does he want to die?"

These people didn't have bad intentions—they truly meant well. They just didn't understand the insidiousness of the disease. And this is even more true when the victim is male. During all of the years when we were searching for help, we only found *two* facilities in the entire country that would accept males into residential treatment for eating disorders. On top of that—try getting an insurance company to cover $850 a *day* to "feed someone." It seems outrageous to them.

If you're lucky enough to surmount these challenges, find a spot at a residential treatment center (they always have a waiting list), and figure out how to cover the cost, you are still facing the consequences of taking your child out of his life for three months. You are forcing him to miss school, social activities and his family—everything he cares about and enjoys. And you're exposing him to potential ridicule by unfeeling peers.

But of course the biggest challenge of all remains: He probably doesn't *want* the help you are providing, doesn't want to go into treatment, and once there, doesn't want to stay.

The process of trying to help TJ began as a nightmare, continued to be a nightmare for eight-and-a-half years, and ended worse than any nightmare I could have imagined.

4

Fears Confirmed

SEEING TJ ACCOMPLISH so much and reading the essays he wrote about himself gave us a false sense of well-being; it didn't come close to giving us insight into what he was truly feeling. At the end of his senior year, though, his behavior changed. His phone stopped ringing constantly. He would come home from school and go immediately up to his bedroom and stay for hours doing homework. If he did anything fun, it was with me.

We knew that, at his age, this wasn't normal. Most guys would rather spend their free time with their buddies, not their moms. I loved that TJ and I were so close but my husband reminded me that this wasn't the norm. I rationalized it; after all, we enjoyed so many of the same things. We both loved to play tennis, for instance, and I could give him a pretty good game, since I played competitive tennis. I realize now that he was hiding from the normal social activities he might have participated in because they often revolved around food.

All through high school, TJ continued to get straight A's—in honors courses—and remained involved in sports. He went to all the school dances with a variety of girls. He kept himself so busy that his excuses for not hanging out with his friends very often seemed quite believable. He was too busy accomplishing things! Here's a list of distinctions racked up by TJ in high school:

- National Honor Society
- Michigan Merit Award
- Senior Athletic Award (cross-country, skiing, tennis)
- Okemos High School Award of Appreciation (exemplifying qualities in character that are an asset to the community of OHS)
- President's Education Award for Outstanding Academic Excellence
- Capital Circuit Academic All-League Award
- Michigan Competitive Scholarship
- The Michigan High School Athletic Association Scholar/Athlete Award
- Ann Lohman Good Sportsmanship Scholarship
- State Winner of the Discover Card Tribute Scholarship
- Albion College Presidential Recognition Scholarship
- Two Certificates of Special Congressional Recognition (nominations to the U.S. Air Force Academy and U.S. Naval Academy)

He was playing the game very well at this point. We were diligent about his weigh-ins and made sure he saw his therapist every other week—but somehow, we knew this wasn't "fixing" him.

A tennis friend of mine was fond of saying that TJ was "quick as a cat." As a junior, he had a 12–0 tennis record. During one tournament in his senior year, I was watching him from the bleachers and I noticed that all the other guys were in shorts, even though it was a chilly day. TJ had on winter sweats, a couple of tee shirts, a hooded sweatshirt, and a ski hat. I wondered how he could even move. About halfway through the first set, TJ's opponent hit the ball into his court but TJ barely moved and missed it. I distinctly remember thinking, "Oh, my gosh, he could have *easily* gotten to that ball." I didn't realize that because he hadn't eaten all day, he had simply run out of energy by 4:30 in the afternoon.

I worried about TJ, of course, but I wondered if I was overreacting. After all, not one of TJ's teachers, coaches or friends had said one word to me about his condition. After TJ died, I went back to his running coach and warned him to please be aware of eating disorders—in the boys as well as the girls. He was naturally distraught and guilt-ridden. He had loved TJ.

"Susan," he said, "never once did it enter my mind that he could have this problem. I always thought that if any of my kids would run a marathon, it would be TJ. He was just so disciplined and motivated. I thought he ran so often and so hard because he wanted to better himself."

The coach wasn't alone; everyone thought that. In those days, TJ was already an expert at hiding his illness.

We may not have understood what was happening to TJ at the time, but he clearly did—at least when he looked back on it in 2003. Here's how TJ expressed it in his journal. His Christmas-light analogy is particularly vivid, showing what a good writer he was, and how carefully he thought about things.

Just because I was losing weight or not gaining, by no means does that signify what I wanted. This is a common misconception towards individuals with eating disorders. A large number of anorexics have no intention of losing weight or being dangerously thin, despite all of the signs that point to that. In a way that is why the disorder is easy to cover up. I always had a supply of protein powder for muscle gain. I lifted weights four times each week. They say that the meal immediately after lifting weights is the most crucial for muscle growth and recovery. I would always have a very large, healthy and balanced meal after lifting weights. It was always accompanied by a hardy protein shake. However, it was then followed up by long periods of not eating. I could not help it. I told everybody that I was trying to put on muscle weight. I lifted and I drank muscle gain drinks—how could I be anorexic? The meals after working out were the only healthy meals that I was having for a while. I was only fooling myself by believing that one big meal after lifting would actually build muscle mass. I honestly wanted to put on muscle weight—but only that. I was not willing to put on any fat at all, under any circumstance.

My eating disorder was on and off during high school. It was comparable to Christmas lights—in the daylight they are barely noticeable, but once darkness sets in, they are impossible to miss. Many people fail to realize the main concept and catch with eating disorders; food is not always the main issue! I was never afraid of food.

It became increasingly difficult to watch what TJ was eating. He wouldn't put anything into his mouth that had any fat in it; it had to say "o grams of fat" on the label. He somehow managed to keep his weight at 110 while eating food that had zero fat, because at that point, he was still consuming calories. I would glance at him out of the corner of my eye when I was at the kitchen table. He would open the refrigerator, eat some carrots and then spray zero-fat butter spray in his mouth. He would eat plates full of the same foods: celery, zero-fat cottage cheese, zero-fat bread, carrots, and egg whites. He would constantly chew gum because he read that it burned calories. He would stand up whenever possible for the same reason.

Each night, we sat down as a family to eat dinner and I would yell upstairs, "TJ! Dinner is ready, honey." The three of us would hear "pound, pound, pound" on the floor: He was making himself do a *thousand* sit-ups before he could eat.

One particular night he came down and said, "I'm not eating here tonight, Mom. I am going to Adam's house for a team dinner before our big match tomorrow."

John and Jessie rolled their eyes as if to say, "Yeah, right."

"Oh, OK, Teej," I replied. "Have a great time. Say hi to Adam's mom for me."

With a, "'Bye guys!" he was off.

I waited two minutes, grabbed my keys and said, "I'll be right back." I went to Adam's house and was so relieved when I saw his street lined with cars and pickup trucks. They really *were* having a team dinner! I looked around, but no white pickup. Following my instinct but dreading what I'd find, I drove over to our local athletic club. My heart sank when I spotted TJ's truck. I went inside and peeked through the window into the workout area and saw him frantically running on the treadmill.

Many times after that day, it was the same scenario: I would follow him to the club and drag him out (or ask the management to kick him out), only to find that he'd driven to another club and snuck in. I even took his picture into that club and said, "He is *not* allowed to work out here. He is not healthy enough. If his heart stops while he's in here, I will hold you liable." I told them about the

time that TJ was lifting weights at 6 in the morning with
no one around to spot him. He'd dropped a heavy weight
on his neck and couldn't lift it off. When he'd told me
about it, I'd asked him how he'd gotten it off.

"I don't know, Mom," he told me. "It was weird. It just
kind of lifted off."

"TJ, how many times can God save your life before
you listen to Him?"

When TJ's senior pictures arrived, the first thing he asked
me was, "Mom, do I look too skinny?" He didn't want to
look skinny—he wanted to have muscles. But the obsession with avoiding all fat was making that impossible.

Don't think I didn't explain that to him. I talked until I
was blue in the face about it, insisting that you can't have
muscles if you don't have something to make muscles out
of! I even tried getting him a personal trainer for a month
because he said he would do what it took to gain weight
as long as it was all muscle and not fat. He mastered every
exercise she gave him and added it to his repertoire, but
ate none of the food she advised him to eat.

Then I got devious. I would sneak into the kitchen at
one in the morning to switch his zero-fat Pringles with
the regular kind. I would add extra oil to our stir-fry
meals. I bought him zero-fat Edy's ice cream, figuring
that at least he was eating calories.

One day I came home and caught my husband crawl-
ing up the basement stairs with a big black garbage bag
in his teeth. (His multiple sclerosis prevents him from
walking.) Rivulets of some liquid were oozing out of a
small tear in the bag, making a dark smear all the way up
the beige carpeting that lined the steps as John climbed.

He had crawled down a full flight of stairs, laboriously made his way across the basement floor, and taken all of TJ's fat-free food out of his "stash" and refrigerator.

"What are you doing?" I shrieked.

He dropped the bag in front of him so he could answer. "This is all going in the trash," he said firmly, catching his breath. "We can't allow fat-free food in this house any longer! It's like putting alcohol in a house with an alcoholic!"

"John, I'm so afraid that if he doesn't eat this food—he won't eat *anything*!" I pleaded.

Silently, he got into his wheelchair and carried the trash bag to the dumpster down the street. I followed him a few minutes later and dug through the garbage until I found the bag, brought it home, and put all of TJ's food back where it came from. I honestly thought I was losing my mind.

John didn't say a word. We were desperate, but neither of us knew what to do—and it seemed as if no one else had any answers, either.

In the spring of TJ's senior year, with a month left until graduation, his therapist informed me that he had consulted with his peers in California, where male eating disorders were more prevalent.

"They are finding little success with curing males," he told me. "I really think TJ should be in a hospital."

I sat there in shock. I was trying to absorb what he'd said first—that there really isn't much hope—and then the idea of putting TJ in the hospital with *four weeks* left of his senior year!

"I . . . I'm very uncomfortable with what you're suggesting," I told him. "TJ has worked *so* hard and I want him to be able to graduate with his friends! How could I do that to him? He doesn't deserve it!"

We talked it through and I agreed to the hospitalization,

but suggested that we wait the four weeks. After all, what was four weeks when the therapist had been working with him for *four years*?!

"Mrs. Barry, it's your choice—but I want you to understand how serious this is. His condition is such that if he were driving in a car with his buddies and a gust of wind came through the open window, his heart could stop."

I stared at him, numb.

I told my family about the plan but the four subsequent weeks were excruciating. Every time he left the house, I felt panic-stricken. Every time the phone rang, I held my breath. Three more weeks . . . two more weeks . . . one more week. . . . Please God, let him be OK.

I had every intention of following through on getting him into the hospital, but his godparents, Ken and Linda, were planning an intervention to make sure it happened. They were afraid that it would be too emotionally draining for me to handle alone, when TJ and I were so close and he could be so persuasive. The two of them and his Uncle Jerry planned the intervention without sharing the specifics with any of us.

We all went to his graduation. He looked horribly thin, very unhealthy, though he appeared to be happy. He posed for pictures with his friends and all of us, and we were about to head back to our house for a party.

"Hey, TJ," my brother called out. "Come here and talk to me for a second."

TJ obediently followed—and before he knew what was happening, they'd grabbed him and locked him in the van, informing him that he was going to the hospital. I watched in disbelief.

It was one of the worst days of our lives. Apparently TJ screamed and cried the entire way to the hospital, pleading with his godparents to let him go. At home, not knowing what was going on, I wept openly for hours, even though I had a house full of guests. Linda had been determined to get him help, even knowing that he'd fight it every step of the way. She told anyone who would listen to her that she would not leave until someone agreed to help him.

There was just one problem: By this time, TJ was 18 ... not a good age for intervention. Short of having him declared incompetent and becoming his custodians, we really had no rights as parents to make decisions for our child anymore.

Linda fought like a mother bear for TJ. She refused to leave the hospital until they agreed to help him. Thanks to her perseverance, he was admitted to an eating disorder program with six or eight women. They managed to hold on to him for 16 days—though he complained bitterly and insisted to me that it wasn't much of a "program"— more of a "unit full of crazy women."

But when the 16 days were up, the doctor in charge (well known in his field) called me and said, "Mrs. Barry, you need to come get your son."

"*What*?!"

"He is 18 and he doesn't want to be here, so we must release him."

All of that effort and trauma for 16 days? TJ was no better off than when he went in—in fact, we were all a bit worse for wear.

Later, TJ wrote:

I skipped high school. All four years of it. Sure, I was around here and there from time to time. I had a lot of fun, too. Hundreds of friends, everybody knew me, always doing something or going someplace. I received awards, scholarships, a 3.93 GPA, and sports recognition. Nonetheless, I missed out on high school. I was lying to myself the entire time. However, ask anybody at my school and they would have told you that TJ had everything going for him without a worry in his life. The girls loved him, he was cool with all the guys, drove a brand new truck—he had it going on. High school was a fake. I hid my disease from absolutely everybody. Anytime something was brought up, I could easily find a way to sugarcoat it and prove that there was nothing wrong. If my friends knew about the eating disorder, I do not think I would have suffered so immensely from it. When I was hiding it from them, I would get caught up in so many lies that it all contributed to my disease. Each lie I made just enabled me to go further into my disorder. Had my friends and acquaintances known however, they surely would have confronted me about my actions when they noticed them.

A subsequent journal entry shows how the many lies he told started coming easily to him. There was nothing he wouldn't do or say to protect the illness.

It was a blizzard outside, 5 degrees below zero and over 15 inches of snow. My parents were getting ready for work when I assured them I was headed to the sledding hill. When I returned home my mom asked, "Are you meaning to tell me that you just got back from sledding for five hours with your friends and you're wearing warm ups?"

"Swear I was. It wasn't too cold once we started sledding."

"That's it . . . no truck for a week. No working out. No tennis. No sit-ups. No nothing."

Work had been cancelled for virtually every business in the area. How could I have been so naive to think that my parents would have to go to work in such conditions? They had gone to every single bump in the landscape that could possibly have resembled a sledding hill. They had called over 25 of my friends' parents (my friends were all still sound asleep). Above all, they had seen my pick up at a fitness club. I came home to find them at the door with tears freezing down my mom's worried cheeks.

Truth be told, I had gone running for one hour in the blizzard, done sit ups for another hour, lifted weights for two and a half hours, and played a half hour of basketball. I did not have breakfast. My parents knew I had lied to their faces and gone to work out. I continued to deny it: I went with friends that they didn't call; we just met at the club and I got a ride with my friend to the hill; we were probably on the other side of the hill so you didn't see us. I had been caught. We all knew it, but I would not admit to it.

Later that day a bunch of friends called to go sledding—I had "already gone." I spent the day doing homework and feeling sorry for myself. It killed me when my parents wouldn't even let me shovel my elderly neighbor's driveway for her. My mom shoveled it all by herself, and it made me the most jealous person alive. She got all that exercise and fresh air while I sat inside.

Such instances went from happening once a year, to once a month, to once every couple weeks, to once a week, to once every couple days. I thought I was in total control. I was eating and exercising how I wanted and when I wanted. I believed that everybody else was jealous. Most people just have one motive or reason behind their actions or just one form of dealing with it. However, throughout my four high school years, the disease took on many forms. At the beginning, it was in fact the textbook definition of anorexia. I would skip meals with the intent of losing weight and having a flatter stomach. Many hours were spent looking at the clock: "Just 14 more minutes until 12 o'clock and then I will have skipped breakfast and have lunch." Many sick thoughts like that ran through my mind day after day. While I was restricting my intake of food, I was not over-exercising in the beginning. That drastically changed.

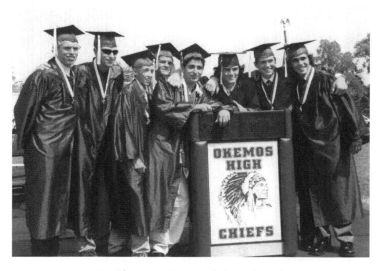

Graduation Day with best friends

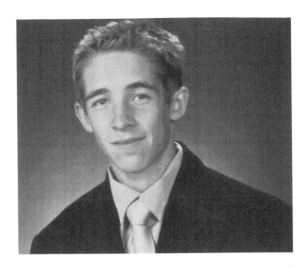

Senior Pictures

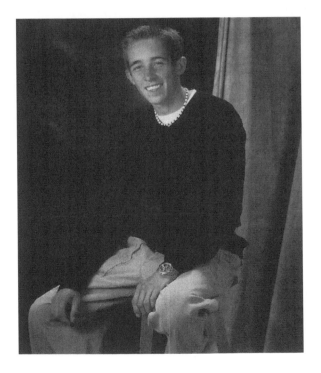

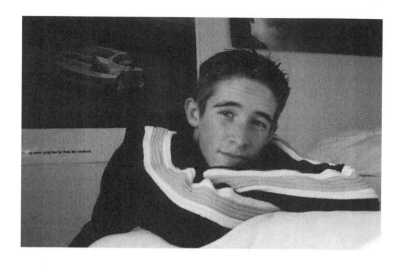

Spring of junior year

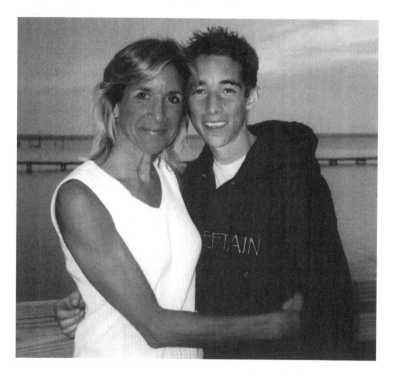

Spring of Senior Year

5

College Years: From Bad to Worse

TJ's UNCLE JERRY had gone to the Naval Academy, and TJ realized that following in his footsteps could provide him with a top-notch education, compliments of our government. The best education and money in the bank—two things that were right up TJ's alley! After many outstanding letters of recommendation were written on TJ's behalf, Congressman Mike Rogers nominated him for admission. Everything was in order academically and in regard to his character, and he even passed all of the physical fitness tests. Actually, he did have trouble with one, involving throwing a ball from the kneeling position. I remember standing in the window watching him practice over and over until he mastered it.

There was only one last thing to pass: his physical. I was very worried about that one. These guys are very smart, I thought. They are going to take one look at TJ and know he has a problem. Imagine my surprise when he came home and told me that he'd passed with flying colors.

Later that day, I went into his room and saw the Air Force Academy folder on his bed. I leafed through the contents until I found the form with all of his vitals, measurements, weight, etc. The minimum weight requirement was 107. I found TJ's weight filled in on the form: *exactly* 107. He'd done it again. He was exactly the weight he needed to be, but not one ounce more.

TJ waited all summer for news, letting the University of Michigan and Michigan State University acceptance letters sit past their deadlines without responding to them. He was confident that he'd end up where he wanted to be.

Finally, one late summer day, the letter from the Air Force Academy arrived. He was so excited. Even though he knew that his dad and I were not on speaking terms, he asked if I would drive with him to Williamston so we would both be with him when he opened it. He wanted us both there to be proud of him.

Of course I did as he wished. When we were all together, TJ opened the envelope very carefully, to preserve this cherished souvenir.

The letter started: "We unfortunately cannot offer you acceptance . . ."

TJ stopped reading, put the letter back in the envelope, stood up and said, "Let's go, Mom."

No one said a word. We drove home in silence. For once in my life, I could not think of anything to say that would make everything okay. TJ's heart broke that night. Mine shattered. Neither of us could believe he hadn't been accepted, so I called to ask why not. I was told that he failed to meet the "minimum seated height requirement."

We had to move on to Plan B—and quickly. TJ was leaning toward U of M, although he was a true MSU Spartan fan at heart. I tried to convince him to go to Albion, a small private college 45 minutes away from home. I wanted him where someone could keep an eye on his health, where people would know his name, where he'd be in small classes and not swallowed up by a huge university.

Albion gave TJ a $10,000 Presidential Scholarship based on his grades—making it easy choice. Then TJ got on the Internet, wrote some essays and earned a few more thousand dollars. Welcome to Albion.

He and his cousin Rhett had grown up together and were very close. They were the same age and had much in common. They both were smart, driven, athletic, cute, popular, and well-liked. They had often talked and dreamed about rooming together in college and, amazingly, this came to fruition. Rhett was going to Albion to play football. TJ wanted to play on the tennis team and run track. What a perfect plan! At least, that is what we hoped.

TJ wanted a single room and we allowed it. *Big mistake.* It wasn't because he wanted a quiet environment in which to study, as he told everyone. It was so that he would have a place to hide: to hide how he looked, the small amount he ate, and the fact that he exercised four hours a day.

He also insisted on an extremely demanding schedule of classes, which gave him yet another perfect excuse to stay in his room. He had to get special permission to enroll in three lab classes (organic chemistry, inorganic chemistry and biochemistry) along with his other studies.

Rhett told us later that he used to knock on TJ's dorm-room door, and he knew TJ was in there, but TJ would stay quiet, pretending he wasn't there. Clearly, he was embarrassed about his physical appearance and unwilling to engage in any social activities that might involve food and drink.

The tennis and track teams did not work out for TJ. I talked to both coaches and told them the truth about his anorexia. I insisted that, at his doctor's orders, he not be permitted to participate in either sport unless he

maintained a marginally healthy weight of 110 pounds—
far more than he weighed at that time. The track coach
kindly said that he would still let TJ come to the meets.
He hoped maybe that would motivate him to gain weight.
I asked him to say "motivate him to get healthy" rather
than "motivate him to gain weight."

The coach told me that after one meet, the team stopped
at Burger King to grab some dinner. TJ pretended to be
asleep. Several of his teammates tried to wake him up,
but he appeared to be in a deep sleep. They left him on
the bus while they all went to order their meals. When I
heard this, I knew TJ hadn't been sleeping. I also knew he
could have won an Academy Award for his performance.

6

Enough Is Enough

In sheer desperation, I decided to go right to the top administrator at the college. I emailed the president and pleaded with him to go to TJ's dorm, knock on his door, and advise him to seek help. I warned that it was very possible that someone would find my son dead on the floor of his room if he didn't take action—and pointed out that this was not the kind of publicity he would want. The email I got back from him will forever be burned into my memory.

> Dear Mrs. Barry, Please know that Albion College has been, is, and will continue to act in TJ's best interest.

What's worse, the school saw fit to forward the whole exchange to TJ—to which he responded to me, angrily, "Unbelievable . . . just mind-boggling."

I emailed the president back.

> Good morning. I received this email from TJ last night after his appointment with Dr. D. He was irate with me for writing to you. I find it totally appalling and unprofessional that a letter that I wrote to you would be shared with TJ by Dr. D. Where are MY privacy rights?

Again, I felt so frustrated, so alone in this battle to save my son's life. I just wanted to scream as loudly as I could for as long as I could.

By the middle of TJ's first term at Albion, we knew it was time to take decisive action. We told him he had to go to a residential treatment center. The therapists just weren't making a difference and he appeared to be getting worse. We informed him that we'd withdraw our financial support for college if he didn't go for the treatment.

Because TJ was not about to spend his own hard-earned money, and because we remained strong and insistent, he conceded. This was what I believe to have been the first of many little miracles in our journey. Looking back, I still can't believe he agreed to leave in the middle of his first term.

TJ was a devout and rigid schedule-follower and we wanted to do what we could to provide him some continuity. We made several pleading, tearful phone calls, begging both the treatment center and his college professors to allow him to complete his classes online while he was in residential. The people at Albion were wonderfully cooperative in communicating to TJ that his health was the most important thing and that his classes would still be there for him when he was well.

Another challenge in getting help for a loved one suffering from an eating disorder is convincing him to make "the phone call." A prospective patient over the age of 18 has to call the treatment facility himself and say that he *wants* to go to residential. The very nature of the illness makes it hard—if not impossible—for him to feel this way or express it. A plea for help just will not leave the mouth of an anorexic. He doesn't want help. He doesn't think he needs it.

This makes his family's attempts to get him to residential treatment terrifying and nearly insurmountably difficult. First, getting him to make the call usually involves bribery or outright force. Second, his school needs to cooperate. (Many young people facing this are in college and have already paid for and started classes.) Third, battling the insurance companies is a nightmare. Many don't cover residential stays at all; others cover only part of the cost—for a brief period of time or until the patient reaches a certain weight. Rarely is that enough—though, in fairness, mental health parity laws have recently improved coverage for psychological illnesses.

The price of residential treatment is outrageous, ranging anywhere from $500 to $1,500 a day. That puts it out of reach for many who need help but can't navigate the insurance labyrinth. And finally, if he does get there, the patient has "privacy rights" preventing parents from accessing any information their child doesn't want them to have. This is in spite of the fact that it is usually the parents who are paying for the treatment—sometimes by draining their savings or even refinancing their homes.

Then, there are the lies. My son never told even a little white lie as a child. Once he developed anorexia, we could never believe a word he said on the subjects of food, exercise or weight. So . . . we couldn't get information from the medical establishment and we couldn't get honest answers from TJ! We found ourselves fighting both the system and our own precious child. Sadly, this is quite typical.

Of course, I understand the thinking behind wanting the patient to make the call. Therapy can't be truly effective unless he *wants* to get well and is willing to make a commitment to the treatment. But when a young person is severely malnourished—starving to death—his brain isn't functioning properly. He becomes trapped in a downward spiral from which he is incapable of breaking free on his own. At that crucial point, it may be necessary to apply pressure. In TJ's case, that is exactly what I did.

I strongly believe that once an anorexic falls below a certain weight, it is as if a toilet has been flushed. You cannot stop the force of it once you've pulled the handle. He starts going down the drain and no matter what you say, how much he seems to understand or how miserable he becomes, he cannot stop the behavior that is killing him. This is what most parents fail to understand until it is too late. They think if they switch therapists or engage a dietician or just say the right thing, something will "click" and their child will start eating again. If only that were true.

Michigan has no residential treatment centers that accept male patients—so my mother, TJ's stepmother Barbara, and I set off on the long trip to pick TJ up at college and drive across a few states to Wisconsin. From the minute we arrived at Albion, we were impatient to get on the expressway heading out of Michigan—but we had to get him on board first. When we arrived at his dorm, TJ gave us his remaining coupons for "free food" at the student snack bar and suggested we go get some lunch while he "tied up some loose ends." My mom and Barbara shot me a look as if to say, "Do not let him leave!"

"Ok, honey," I said to him, smiling casually. "Take your time with what you need to do, and we'll go get some lunch. How about half an hour?"

He agreed, and we parted. As soon as he was out of hearing range, my cohorts were frantic. "Susan! He is not coming back! Why did you let him go?"

"I have to trust him," I said.

We came back at the agreed-upon time and he was not

there. My heart sank but I pretended to be unfazed and said, "Just chill you two. We can wait." A minute later, he came in the door and I heaved a silent sigh of relief.

We got in the car and as we headed off campus, TJ yelled, "Stop the car, Mom!"

"What is it, TJ?" I asked, thinking that he'd forgotten something. As I pulled over and slowed down, he opened the door, jumped out and started to run.

Again, panic from moms and Grandma. We sat there, stunned and frozen. He ran until he caught up with one of his professors, on her way to teach a class. They exchanged words and then TJ jogged back to the car. He told us he'd wanted to know if she had finished grading his exam from the day before.

Needless to say, I was relieved when we finally got on the expressway—but I still worried that he'd find a way to run or that he'd change his mind or pass out. We arrived at Rogers Memorial Hospital in Oconomowoc, Wisconsin, in about six hours, and TJ did a great job of navigating us right up the driveway to the front entrance. Surprisingly, he was in pretty good spirits.

An administrator immediately took us on a tour. It was a beautiful place that looked like a big ski lodge near a pretty lake. As our guide showed us the dining room, he pointed out the toasters, hidden away under a counter. "We put the toasters down here, out of sight," he said.

"Why would you do that?" I asked, genuinely baffled.

"Toasting is actually a behavior we discourage," he told us. "Many eating-disorder patients toast all of their bread because they believe it burns some of the calories out."

He also told us that gum was prohibited because many anorexics chew it to replace the satisfaction of eating—and because they believe that chewing gum burns calories. (When TJ's suitcase was checked during admittance,

several packs were ferreted out and confiscated.) Later,
TJ told me that the patients hide gum above the ceiling
tiles and outside in the bushes. "There are so many tricks,
Mom," he told me, "and these people are extremely smart
at coming up with new ones."

After we'd finished the tour and completed all the necessary paperwork, it was time for the heartbreak of saying
good-bye. TJ hugged each of us in turn. His Grandma
Frances started to cry. When he reached for me, we were
both sobbing and neither one of us wanted to let go.

The first three weeks were horrible. We weren't allowed
much communication. Maybe, I thought, it was like
Marine boot camp, where they break down the recruits
by taking away all control. Or maybe it was to protect
us parents from hearing our kids say how horrible the
place was. They surely didn't want us coming to rescue
our sobbing and pleading kids.

After a month, TJ had gained 10 pounds and pretty much stopped complaining. We occasionally got a
glimpse of the old TJ, who charmed us with his wit and
personality. Hearing him laugh made me happy and
hopeful for days. The best part of having TJ in residential treatment was knowing he was safe; that someone
else was responsible for his well-being. I could sleep
again. The phone could ring without my heart skipping
a beat. He was eating and gaining weight. Our insurance
company was paying $850 a day to feed our son. I was
so incredibly grateful that I took the insurance woman I
spoke with on the phone out to lunch!

TJ had filled out questionnaires designed to deter-
mine whether he was obsessive-compulsive or battling
depression. He passed both tests with flying colors—the
therapists didn't see signs of OCD. Then I realized that he
must have worked hard to fill in answers that would yield

a clean bill of mental health. He'd been able to outsmart the test! No one can tell me that a normal male teenager has everything lined up and ready for the next day by 4:30 each afternoon.

At Rogers, everything revolves around a color system and rewards are based on the color each patient attains by gaining weight. TJ started at the red level. He wasn't allowed to walk even as far as the next building, just yards away; he had to ride in a van. Gradually, he progressed to the yellow level, then green. At each new color stage, he was given additional privileges.

TJ was motivated to earn the right to go on a putt-putt golf outing, go fishing on the lake, go to the mall, to the movies, bowling, and even to a Milwaukee baseball game. He loved sports and competition so this system worked for him. By the second month, he had gained *20 pounds* and seemed happy.

Very little was explained to me by the staff at Rogers, but a former patient there described the stages to me as follows:

Observation Level—Patient's first 72 hours, under strict supervision, cannot leave the building.

Red level—Significantly underweight, no physical activities (not even walking), no passes off premises (also, if concerns exist over self-mutilation or running away).

Yellow level—The patient making good progress! May be close to or at goal weight, not engaged in eating disorder behavior, and is opening up in groups. Can begin physical activity, go on daily walks, take part in weekly outings such as miniature golf, and get "off-ground" passes much more easily and for longer periods of time.

Green level—Nearing discharge, at goal weight, can use the weight room. Trust is being formed between patient and treatment team. Can even take walks solo, with no supervision, and can get passes to leave all day or for the weekend.

He went on to tell me that levels can be revoked at any time. If a patient starts losing weight or ceases to comply with his meal plan, he can be dropped back down to yellow or red.

TJ recognized the bizarre behaviors of the other patients. He would tell me how he was helping everyone else. He said he had talked privately and prayed with one boy who would "throw up in his mouth" at the dinner table. He'd cheer up the sad one, play games with the lonely one. He told me about one boy who was compelled to do everything eight times—open the door, flush the toilet, turn on the light, wash his hands, etc. TJ was quick to recognize everyone else's problems and wanted to help them all. I wondered who was helping TJ.

In the beginning, TJ got caught doing sit-ups in his room, hiding banana bread in the hood of his sweatshirt at dinner, spewing food into his napkin when he "sneezed," hiding food in his pockets and then dumping it over the balcony. According to him, there was a huge pile of food on the ground beneath the balconies, the result of widespread dumping on the part of residents. (Rogers must have had the happiest squirrel population on the planet!)

In one phone conversation, TJ told me he got up in the middle of the night to go to the bathroom and discovered a 12-year-old boy, new to the program, running in place in the washroom at 2 in the morning! When TJ walked out of the bathroom, he spotted one of the counselors looking out the window.

"What are you doing, Steve?" TJ asked, choosing to say nothing about the boy he'd just encountered.

"Come on over here, TJ, sit down," the counselor replied. He had a clipboard and was writing down tally marks. "You see that girl out there? She will run around the house 100 times before she stops exercising."

"Why would anyone do that?" TJ exclaimed. "She'll *never* get out of here."

When he relayed that last part to me in a phone call, I felt my heart sink.

"TJ," I said sharply into the phone, betraying my impatience. "She should stop doing that so that she can get healthy—not in order to get out of treatment!"

It was then that I began to doubt whether TJ was really getting well at all.

Christmas was fast approaching but TJ was scheduled to be at Rogers for another month. One evening, he called and begged me to "come to my senses." He must have known how desperately I wanted to believe he was recovering.

Mom! I've already been here two months and they want me to stay another one! They have to be kidding! I've gained 20 pounds and have been so compliant with everything they have asked me to do! Please. Don't make me be here at Christmas. I want to come home and then start my second semester at Albion. I don't want to miss an entire semester, Mom—it will mess everything up. They only want me here because almost everyone is gone because of the holidays. They just want our money! I get this now, Mom, I really do. I want to stay healthy. I feel great. I promise to gain the last 10 pounds at Albion. I'll make a contract with them and I will sign it. I'll see a therapist every week, a dietician every week, and have my blood drawn every other week. You can call and check to see if I am following through, and I won't be mad. I promise. Please, Mom, please. Don't make me miss Christmas at home. You know how much I love Christmas. No one will be left here. Everyone is going home, and they won't even have any normal groups or therapy.

If you are a parent, you can relate to how much I wanted to believe everything TJ said in that phone call—but I stood firm. I told him I wasn't going to bring him home against medical advice. He started to cry and hung up. I'm not sure which of us was in the most pain at that moment.

7

Live And Learn

THE FIRST TIME through residential treatment, we made a major mistake. We believed that by the end of it, he'd actually gotten well. After the first two months and a weight gain of 20 pounds, he seemed to be on his way back to his normal self, and he certainly said all the right words. Even still, I didn't let TJ come home for Christmas. I stayed strong, rebuffed his pleas, and followed Rogers' recommendation. It nearly killed me to keep TJ away from home at holiday time, but I explained to him that it was because I wanted him home for many Christmases to come.

I did, however, relent about school: I let him come home in time to start his second semester in January. He had been in residential treatment from October 24th, 2002, until January 9, 2003. He was admitted at 85 pounds and was released at 106—a gain of 21 pounds. That sounds like a substantial amount, but at 20 years old and a stunted 5 feet 5 inches tall, 106 is still far from normal. TJ agreed to sign a contract stating that he'd continue to gain, so we reluctantly arranged for him to be released a few weeks early.

There was a lot of stress in the air when he came home. None of us felt certain how to act around him, what to say, what not to say. "You look great" might be interpreted as, "You've gained weight," and we weren't sure he'd react well to hearing that.

We wondered how closely we should monitor his meals. Should we insist he continue to eat three meals and two snacks a day, as he had in treatment? What if he didn't comply? What if he wanted fat-free food? How much exercise was permissible? Would it be all right for me to go for a run with him or must I say not yet? Who was going to weigh him? What if he started losing weight?

They'd told us to throw away the scale (as if he wouldn't find another). They told us to throw away his skinny clothes and buy him bigger ones (unnecessary, because now the clothes he'd been swimming in actually fit). That was nearly all the advice we got, other than to follow up with a counselor and a dietician. I felt we should have had some additional training before his release.

Interestingly, I felt some of the same apprehensiveness I'd experienced when I brought TJ home as a newborn. I remember standing at my kitchen window with that impossibly tiny infant in my arms, waiting for my mom to drive up the driveway and teach me what to do with him! I felt equally helpless now.

TJ lived up to the terms of his contract for the most part. He agreed to see a therapist weekly, but insisted that he didn't need a dietician because he knew as much as they did about what he needed to eat: He had it all memorized. I agreed. He did know what he needed to do. Getting himself to *do* it was the challenge. He agreed not to exercise until he'd gained his final pounds. It all sounded good. We were "cautiously optimistic."

The weekend before he went back to college was hard. I was so happy to see how good he looked, although his food intake wasn't what I wanted it to be. I remember watching the clock: noon . . . 1 . . . 1:30 . . . 2. . . . Finally, I'd say, "TJ, aren't you going to have lunch?"

"Mom, I had a big breakfast," he'd reply. "I'm not

hungry yet. Besides, you and Jess haven't eaten lunch either!"

"TJ, that's because we just ate breakfast two hours ago! You had breakfast three hours before we even got up!"

"Mom, you have to trust me. Don't worry about me, OK? I don't want to be watched."

He wanted to play tennis with me. He wanted to go for a run with me. I felt I just couldn't allow that until he gained those last 10 promised pounds and hit the minimum goal weight Rogers had set for him. I did go for walks with him, taking that opportunity to encourage him to keep gaining so he could be physically active again.

I took TJ back to Albion on schedule, just a day before the start of classes. After a few big hugs and many reassurances from him that he'd be fine, I watched him climb the steps and disappear inside his building.

One day a few weeks later, I surprised him and drove to school to take him out to dinner. I had been so afraid to let him go back to his single dorm room. Looking back on it, I know that we never should have allowed him to live alone. A roommate could have kept an eye on him and informed us if he wasn't doing well. But he had somehow convinced us, and the university, that he needed a single room.

At his urging, we decided to eat at the cafeteria. As we left, I was surprised to see TJ take handfuls of fresh fruit with him. I knew that was not allowed. When I asked him about it, he mumbled something about it being fine. (I believe he had gotten a "504 deviation," which allows someone with a disability or health issue to operate outside of an institution's rules. For example, because of my husband John's multiple sclerosis, he gets extremely overheated. When he filed a 504, his school district installed an air-conditioning unit in his classroom, though none of the other teachers could have one.)

I learned that every Monday, TJ went directly to the cafeteria's kitchen. He'd forged a wonderful friendship with the cook, Phyllis, and she had become his favorite person at Albion. She always beamed when he walked in, and yelled, "Thomas!!" She would have a dozen hard-boiled eggs ready for him, which he would take back to his room. What she didn't know was that he'd systematically throw out the yolks and eat just the whites. Phyllis liked to tell TJ that when he became a dentist, he would owe her some gold fillings.

Counselors at Albion offered to send TJ to Ann Arbor regularly, in the school van, to see an eating disorder specialist. I thought this was incredible, but for some reason, he only went a few times. I never knew why and they weren't permitted to enlighten me: Those privacy rights intervened again.

Every other weekend, TJ came home—with his laundry, of course! We would always go to Baskin Robbins, where he'd get fat-free ice cream and I'd get Pralines and Cream. We would walk around Michigan State University's campus and he would work his way through a written list of things he wanted to tell me or ask me. As we covered each topic, he would cross it off his list. I tried to think of it as cute, how organized and time-efficient my son was. Deep down, I knew better.

He loved to hear news of the family—all about his cousins, aunts, uncles, and grandparents, as well as his friends. We didn't talk about food or weight except for a quick, "How are you doing, honey?"

I always got the same answer: "I'm good, Mom."

After one weekend visit, he left this note on my bed:

FOOD TO BRING ME AT COLLEGE!
(Welcome at every visit!)
Butter spray
Jimmy John's bread (as much as you can get!)
Carrots
Fat-free Pringles
Rice cakes
Celery
Sugar-free/fat-free candy
Sugar-free/fat-free ice cream
Crystal light/Snapple
Fat-free pretzels
Fat-free yogurt
Gum!
Hard-boiled egg whites

TJ'S WELCOME HOME MEALS
Spaghetti dinner—Great Harvest Bread, wheat rolls
Salad—with veggies and fat-free dressing
Fat-free spaghetti sauce
French toast—made with Egg Beaters and skim milk,
    sugar-free syrup, and butter spray
Pancake Supper—fat-free batter, butter spray, sugar-free
    syrup
Omelet—Egg Beaters with fat free cheese and veggies
Scrambled eggs
White rice and veggie stir-fry

One of the most frustrating weekends came just four
weeks after TJ left Rogers. He was looking thinner and
I couldn't get any information about how he was doing, so I was very upset. I didn't think it made any sense

that he had an illness that he couldn't admit to, that our insurance was paying to treat, about which we couldn't find out a thing!

I made TJ tell me what he weighed and he confirmed my fears. Instead of gaining those final 10 pounds, he had *lost* 10. He asked me to help him, to help motivate him, just as the levels had done at Rogers. I could sense his desperation and of course I shared it. I made a deal with him that if he gained five pounds, I would give him $100; if he gained 10 pounds, I would take him on a trip, just the two of us.

Every time TJ walked in the door for one of his weekend visits, I tried to see him clearly and not let my eyes trick me. I wanted so badly to see him looking better. I would say to John, "TJ looks a little better, don't you think?"

His replies varied from, "He looks the same to me," to "How can you tell? He has so many clothes on."

Two weeks after we made our "bargain," TJ came home on a Friday afternoon and, as usual, I tried to sense any change for the better—or worse—in his appearance. I didn't like what I saw. The next morning, he handed me a business envelope.

"What's this?" I asked.

"Read it, Mom."

It was a letter from TJ's therapist at Albion:

Mrs. Susan Barry:

I am writing to you at the request of TJ. Please find enclosed a signed copy of the release of information executed by TJ. It will expire after this weekend. TJ and I have discussed the possibility of initiating mild exercise on the weekends as a means of managing stress and keep-ing emotional balance. TJ has agreed to keep me updated on his exercise and he has also agreed to talk with me if his workouts become problematic for him in terms of compulsive exercise. We have discussed the risks and benefits of this decision. I support TJ's efforts to maintain his physical and emotional health through stress manage-ment and mild exercise. I hope this letter is helpful to you.

I could not believe my eyes! My son was losing weight instead of gaining! How could TJ have talked this "ex-pert" into allowing him to exercise? Didn't he know that there is no such thing as "moderate exercise" to someone like TJ? I knew there was *no way* TJ could maintain a reasonable, healthy exercise regimen!

TJ saw my face and knew I was about to erupt.

"Mom, calm down," he began, before I could even open my mouth. "You're not going to try to come be-tween me and my therapist, are you? You have to trust me, and my therapist, and that he knows what he is doing. OK, Mom? Mom?"

I was speechless. I folded the letter, put it back in the envelope, and handed it back to him. He stood there look-ing at me. I heaved a deep sigh and walked away. A few minutes later, TJ bounded down the stairs in his workout clothes. "I'm going to the gym, OK, Mom?"

I managed a surly, "Have fun."

When TJ left that Sunday, I immediately called his therapist to leave a message on his voice mail.

"Hello, doctor. This is TJ's Mom. TJ showed me the letter of permission for his 'mild' exercise. I do not want you to tell him about this call. He and I are very close and he tells me everything. I am his biggest supporter, and I do not want this to come between us so he feels even more alone in this insidious illness. I think you should know what his 'mild exercise' was. He got up and did one hour of sit-ups—1,000. He ran to and from the gym—four miles. He lifted weights for three hours. He rode the stationary bike for one hour, then did another hour of sit-ups before he left. This was TJ's first day of *mild* exercise. Doctor, I just thought you needed to know this information."

Monday afternoon, TJ called me. "Mom! I can*not* believe you called my therapist!"

I wanted to scream! I could not believe this man—this professional—had betrayed my confidence. How was it possible that TJ had all the "privacy rights" and I had none? Instead of screaming, I just put my head down on the kitchen table and cried. Didn't anybody know how to help him? Didn't anyone understand?

TJ gained five pounds and got the $100 I had promised him. Then he gained another five and we took a five-day cruise to Catalina Island. The amazing dinners on the cruise were terribly stressful. People were eating like kings and queens and loving it. Everyone at our table stared at TJ's plate where, one night sat a plain baked potato and the next, five pieces of shrimp. When TJ wasn't around, I made a point of informing our tablemates that he had an eating disorder. I was getting tired of hiding his condition, pretending everything was normal. I cared that it embarrassed him to talk about it—but his behavior was embarrassing to me; I just couldn't deal with it silently anymore.

In three months, he lost all the weight he had gained. I lost a little more of my mind and another piece of my heart.

8

Tough Love

SHORTLY AFTER HIS latest drastic weight loss, in the spring of 2003, I tried yet another tactic with TJ. Out of sheer desperation I told him that I was done begging and bribing. His stepdad and I were going to have to resort to "tough love." We would not buy or allow in the house any fat-free food. We would gladly purchase food for him if it had at least .5 grams of fat.

Here is the letter I wrote him:

Dear TJ,

I am writing this letter mostly because it hurts too much to look at you and say this all verbally. I am way too emotional right now and on the edge of sanity with worry and frustration over this whole eating disorder ordeal. For the past five years, we have tried everything we thought might help you. Dr. R. was supposed to be the best, four years with him. Dr. S. was supposed to be the best at Beaumont Hospital. Dr. R. was supposed to be the best in the nation. Dr. D. was supposed to be the best and trained in your problem at Albion. We thought we were handing you over to the best. Nothing tried, nothing suggested, nothing demanded has worked. You need to admit that you have a big problem. I think you need to deal with it and fix it yourself. Like Abe Lincoln failing sixteen times in things he tried and ending up being one of the greatest and most successful presidents. Like the guy who had to break his wrist, cut off his own arm and walk eight miles. This will to live. If anyone can conquer this ugly disease you have, it is you. I pray constantly that you will just walk up to me and say, "Mom, I want to try Rogers again. I am going to keep my promise. I said I didn't hate it there and that I would go back if I couldn't gain the last 10 lbs at Albion." TJ, you lost it all. I have trusted, hoped, believed a lot of your words and promises, but there is always an excuse: I didn't have fat-free food, I couldn't exercise, I was being controlled, I wasn't motivated, I was back in the hot seat at Albion, I was mad, I missed all my graduation parties, and on and on. You do what you need to do when the gun is pointed, and as soon as you get what you want, you slide back down. This has happened over and over again. You say you gained three pounds in the last month but you won't let me weigh you. Why should I believe you? Why should I trust you? You said you could gain ten pounds on your own. Didn't. You said you'd go back if you couldn't. Didn't. Fat-free food is not what you need. That is just a Band-aid. What you need is to get your mind fixed so you don't worry about what you told me you're worried about to make you lose all that weight in three weeks. It's not fair to all the people who love you and worry about you and pray so hard for you and cry for you in this state of sadness either. You refuse to take any drug that may help. You refuse to let me see the blood work. You refuse to take vitamins. You refuse to tell me your weight. You want me to ignore it all and trust that you will do what you say. Yet we can all see what you are doing, so your words don't match your actions. . . . at all. At the show tonight, when you all of a sudden slipped back into the theatre we just left, I knew what you were doing. You went back in to hide from Finley and that whole gang, not to visit with them which is what you told us. You know you look bad. . . . that is why you hid. Do you want to act that way the rest of your life—hiding, isolating, lying? That is so not like you. YOU are so not like you. I have tried absolutely everything. I have said absolutely everything. I cannot fix you. It is all up to you, TJ. You have to either hate the way you are living your life so badly or fall over with your heart stopped to scare the crap out of you before you are going to do anything or feel you even need to do anything. I love you but I cannot watch you do this anymore. We will not pay for any more college until you get well. You can work your tail off with dad all summer but will have to use it all to pay for college when we would have. It is your choice. I truly believe you are the only one that can turn your life around and get back to being the TJ we all know and love. I miss that kid sooooo much it makes me sob. Please, please read this letter slowly and think. Consider. Decide. Make this the best day of your life and mine and all the others who love you so much. I love you beyond words.

Mom

I wish I could say that I won this round. After much heated debate, TJ decided that rather than live with my conditions, he would go live with his father, 20 minutes away. We would not speak for two months. During that time, he stopped going to see his therapist at school, prompting the therapist to write him a letter. Here's part of it:

> Dear TJ,
>
> I am contacting you by mail because you have not scheduled an appointment with me yet this semester as per our conversation on December 9, 2003. Your lack of contact with me or the office leads me to conclude that you have decided not to continue counseling here at Counseling Services at this time. I want you to know that this decision is against my clinical judgment. I recommend that you continue to have regular contact with me and with Student Health Services to manage and treat your eating disorder. As we have seen in the past, when you are maintaining regular contact with Counseling Services and Student Health Services, you appear to cope more effectively....
>
> It is important to note that not continuing counseling may be in violation of your signed agreement, dated October 2, 2003, with the VP for Student Affairs and Dean of Students....
>
> Signed,
> Director for Counseling Services

I was miserable and I sensed that TJ was, too—but neither of us would give in. He sent me several emails trying to persuade me to reconsider my position. He told me his dad didn't care if he ate birdseed, as long as he ate. Why couldn't I be like that?

Here's an email I got from him during that time:

Subject: Come on

Mom, I miss you so much. We are missing out on so much. I have so much I want to tell you. Why can't you realize that I am not dying here? I have put on a solid amount of weight, feel great, energized. Just because I don't eat fat? Come on. I can go out to eat places. I can do it. I just don't eat much when I am on my own. Just because it embarrasses you to have me order special requests doesn't mean that you should not pay for college. Is your final answer that you are not paying under any circumstance unless I go to residential? Please answer this question directly.

My response:

TJ, I told you that the isolation, the perfectionism, the control and manipulation, the indecisiveness, the fat phobia, the over-exercising, the inability to spend money, etc., is what is worrisome. It may be helped with a pill. It may be helped in a residential treatment center. It cannot be taken care of by ignoring it. It will not go away. You are choosing not to talk to me, TJ. That isn't coming from me at all. The 15 lbs that you gained is still 15 lbs short of what you were running cross country THREE YEARS ago. You have been hospitalized three times because of your "just like everybody else's weird eating habits." When was the last time you hung out and had fun with friends,

TJ? That is not normal. It doesn't have to be pizza you eat either—you can't even eat .5 grams of fat or low-fat food! That is not normal either, unless you are fat and trying to lose weight. I am not budging on this.

The truth is, this tough-love approach failed horribly and almost resulted in his death.

One day I came home and saw TJ using our lawn mower to cut the neighbors' lawns. I watched him out the window. He seemed so weak, so frail, so terribly thin. It broke my heart. I cried because I was so worried, I missed him, and I felt so guilty. He needed me.

I watched as he finished one lawn and walked across the street to begin a new one—but he couldn't start the mower. He did not have the strength to pull the cord.

Rather than watch him struggle, I went out and joined him and without saying a word, I pulled the cord and started the mower. I said, "I love you, TJ," then went back to my window and watched his progress. To my surprise, he stopped cutting the grass before he was done—very abnormal behavior for TJ. He just got in his truck and left with the lawn half cut! At the time, I didn't understand it, but TJ's account of that evening, as recorded in his journal, explains what happened—and the even more alarming events that followed:

10/22/03
Friday was interesting. Woke up, did my sit-ups (both sets), did my push-up routine (that was from 6 AM to 8 AM), then went to the DOW [student workout center at

Albion] and lifted for two 2 hours. Then I rode the bike for one hour. I went straight to class at 11 AM and was done for the long fall break at 1 PM. I went back to my dorm room, vacuumed, cleaned, packed, did the Torso Trac and some more sit-ups. I left for home at 2 PM. I ate an apple on the way home. I got to dad's and brought in all my stuff. Then I mowed his lawn. I got to the point where it was very hard to walk up the hill. I have mowed lawns for eight years and now could hardly finish one lawn. My legs felt so weak. At first I thought it was just because I had not been exercising my legs very much so they were just out of shape. After mowing, dad came home and we talked for a few minutes before I left to mow lawns in mom's neighborhood. It felt so good to sit down and drive . . . weird! I got to moms and could not pull the mower cord hard enough to start it. Mom had to start the mower. I said, "Thanks," and that was all. I hadn't seen her for probably three weeks. I am not talking to her. She refused to pay for my college because I did not go to the hospital. She and I made a deal for me to gain weight and she would buy me things at certain weights. I gained the weight. She didn't buy them. So anyway, we aren't getting along. I usually run with the mower down the street to the lawns. I could not run. I walked the mower over to the lawn. My legs hurt immediately. I have never felt like that before. My legs were tingling, shaking, weak. I had to stop and rest after every row just to gain the energy to make the next pass. It took me twice as long to mow that lawn. After I finished just the first half of the lawn, I stopped the mower, pretending like it had quit and then acted like it would not start back up again. I had two and a half more lawns to mow—but I just brought it back to

Mom's house. I couldn't finish. I couldn't mow a lawn! Nobody was home when I came in. I hate to waste time. It is my biggest pet peeve. I came in with my list of things to get and do at mom's. I got one thing, read the sports section, and then laid/fell down and lay on the floor for about 15 minutes. I hardly did any of the things I planned on doing when getting there. I told myself I was just going to go to my dad's and sit down and do homework until 9 PM. I was so looking forward to 9 PM all mid-term exam week. I was going to go on the Internet, relax, and have a bunch of food that was at dad's. So I went to Jimmy John's first. Then I would go to dad's. I left my mom's at about 7 PM. I picked up five loaves of day-old bread. I headed home to dad's but did not make it. I didn't get to 9 PM when I planned to enjoy myself and eat.

Apparently, I crashed head on into a lady with a dog in her car at 7:35 PM on Grand River Rd. She was slowing down (5 MPH) getting ready to turn into her neighborhood. I was going 25 MPH. The speed limit was 45 MPH. You know something is wrong when I am going 20 MPH under the limit . . . it's usually the other way! Witnesses say I was driving with my lights off and kept swerving over the curb. I ran over a CATA bus sign, then got back on the road and swerved into the opposing traffic lane where I crashed into the lady's car. I got out of the van and was stumbling around for a while. The police came and I could not respond or even tell him my name. I was taken in an ambulance to Sparrow Hospital.

I awoke to about ten people standing over me in a bed, tubes all over, asking me my name, birth date, parent's name, and phone number. I remember thinking I was in a dream as I lay there. I was not answering their questions because I thought I was dreaming. They kept telling me that I needed to drink some stuff. I wasn't drinking. They said I had to drink it or they would have to stick a tube you-know-where. I drank it. They had me sip it through a straw. It took me forever to finish. They kept saying, "I know it tastes terrible but you need to drink it. I don't remember it tasting like anything.

I had blacked out at the wheel. Normal blood sugar levels are 80–120. My blood sugar was 15, caused by malnutrition and stress. I remember everything that day up to driving to Jimmy John's. I don't recall driving to get the bread or where I parked. I remember trying to get as close as I could. I remember doing a bad parking job and vaguely remember going into Jimmy John's. I was stumbling and looked like an ape or gorilla. My back was hunched over and I was stumbling with each step. My friend, Marco, was working there. He said, "Just take as many as you want." I took five loaves. I kept dropping them on the way to the van although I can't picture it; I just know that I did. From that time until I crashed I only remember these cars flashing their brights at me (my lights were off), and loud sounds of the bottom of the van rubbing up against the curb. I thought I remembered a lady with short hair getting out of her car, looking at it, and shaking her head. I remember screaming three times really loud, "GOSH DARN IT. CONCENTRATE!" when I hit the curb. I had midterm exams the whole week before. I stayed in my room and studied all week. I didn't lift weights or bike, therefore I told myself I didn't need food for energy and I didn't eat much at all. The sad part is—I didn't mind being in that hospital. They gave me heated blankets, an adjustable bed, college football on

TV, remote, free phone, nurses at my service at the press
of a button, any kind of food I wanted, homework . . .

I even told my dad to take his time when picking me up.

The next day, my cousins, Tommy, Jennie, and Carrie,
stopped by my dad's to try to convince me to go back to
Rogers. People called my dad all day. His phone didn't
stop ringing, trying to get him to make me go (people
from my mom's family, too). My mom told everybody.
She exaggerated the situation (she said six signs were
knocked down- actually only one). I have thought about
going to get help, but I am going to give this new Dr. at
the University of Michigan a try. I weigh 75 lbs and have
0% body fat.

Here's my version of that evening, starting with the
phone call no mother wants to receive.

"Mrs. Barry, there has been an accident. Your son TJ
is at Sparrow Hospital. He is okay, but you should come
as soon as you can."

When I got there, TJ was lying on a bed, shaking uncontrollably because he was so cold. They couldn't tell
how old he was. He had IVs hooked up to him and was
white as a ghost. Later, I found out his body temperature
was 89 degrees (normal is 98.6), his heart rate was 32 (normal is 50–100), his blood sugar was 16 (non-conducive to
life), and his liver was liquid-filled. I asked the nurse how
much he weighed. She must have been a mother because
she looked very sad when she replied, "I can't tell you."
I started to cry. She went over to the scale, pressed the
button, and walked away. I could not believe the number
that lit up in red on that scale.

It seemed to us that TJ had hit rock bottom that

night—and we wanted to believe that might be a good thing. Maybe the fact that he'd almost died was a miracle in disguise. People had told me that addicts have to bottom out in order to realize the severity of their situation and change course. We prayed that this was the beginning of TJ's climb out of his illness for good.

I called the hospital the next morning, begging to talk to the doctor caring for TJ. The woman informed me that there were a few doctors in his room right then, consulting with him. I asked if one of them could please call me as soon as that meeting was over.

When the doctor called, I frantically explained to him that I felt we *finally* had TJ in a position where he could be forced to stay in the hospital. The accident proved that he was a danger to himself and others. I was rambling on and on when the doctor finally interrupted me. I'll never forget his words.

"I'm sorry, Mrs. Barry. We just discharged TJ."

I lost it. I yelled into the phone, "Are you serious? Did any of you doctors look under the sheets? How could you possibly release him? He was almost dead 48 hours ago!"

"We don't deal with anorexia here," he told me with icy calm. "We informed TJ of the seriousness of his situation and encouraged him to eat."

Amazingly, TJ was back in class Monday morning.

At this point, too much time had passed with no intervention. He was not getting better and I was desperate. I had tried therapists, dieticians, a personal trainer, bribing rewards, tough love, and finally, the trust that he'd insisted would be the best way to get him to gain weight. (In other words, leave him and his eating disorder alone.)

At his insistence, I pretended to ignore his condition, acting as if everything was fine and showering him with love, support and compliments. This, too, failed miserably.

His father wasn't making him do anything he didn't want to do, and he took over paying for TJ's college. I had nothing to hang over my son's head any longer, no leverage for forcing him back into treatment.

At my wit's end, I went to Community Mental Health and filled out forms and more forms to begin the process of committing TJ to a treatment program against his will. It was a horrendous ordeal, filled with a lot of red tape and waiting.

Finally, the day came when a policeman or two were supposed to come and take TJ away in handcuffs. They informed me they'd take him by surprise in the early evening, while he was working, delivering pizzas.

Naturally, I was a mess all day. In a show of support, good friends of ours we'd confided in had invited us over for dinner to help us bear the stress. We accepted—but right before we were to leave for their house, we got a call from the police saying that they couldn't find TJ.

I was frantic. John and I drove to the pizza place where TJ worked, parked our van down the street, and turned our lights off. A little while later, we saw his car pass ours. Then we saw the police car following his. I told my husband I wanted to leave immediately—I just couldn't bear to watch them handcuff our good and harmless son in front of everyone and drag him off like some criminal. No one there would have a clue why they were taking him. My heart broke in half that night, just imagining his humiliation.

We drove to our friends' house, apologized for being late, and started to play euchre. Honestly, I don't know what I'd have done without their kindness—I was just maxed out, physically and emotionally.

Then my cell phone rang. It was CMH telling me to come get TJ. I could not believe my ears!

When I arrived at the clinic, TJ was waiting to leave. He said, "Mom, that ranked right up there as the dumbest thing you've ever done."

My heart was racing. I had no choice but to let him get in the car. He told me on the way home that they'd asked him only one question: "Do you want to kill yourself?" His reply had been, "Absolutely not. I'm doing great in college. I'm just studying too much and don't have time to eat as well as I should be."

Obviously, they bought it. Or wanted to.

Later, when I calmed down and followed up with a call to CMH, frantically pleading my case and complaining about how the whole thing unfolded, their reply was, "I think we maybe should have handled that differently. If you would like to try again . . ."

Now I want to tell you something very important. If your child is 18 or older and he absolutely refuses to get the help he needs, it is wiser and more efficient to go through the court system. Bring a legal action stating that your child is a danger to himself and others and obtain legal rights over him. Once you are in charge legally, he must do what you tell him to do. He will undoubtedly try to make you feel as if you are the meanest, most awful parents in the world . . . but you can handle that. Let him hate you now so you can love him later. I profoundly wish we'd gone that route, but there is no going back for us.

At the time, I honestly felt I had tried everything. The following is a letter I wrote to him on August 12, 2004, after one year of tough love:

Dear TJ,

We've tried one solid year of tough love to try to convince you that you need residential treatment to turn your life around. We are still certain that is what you need, but we cannot force you. Only you can turn your life around, and I know that taking a few months out of your life seems impossible to you at age 20. The window of opportunity for you to claim back your normal eating and life is closing quickly but nothing anyone can say or do is taken in the way it is meant. You twist everything around, thinking people are against you rather than for you.

There has been some improvement, but it has only been seen for about a month. On July 3rd when you were here, you looked terribly ill. It's a good sign that you bought a car and cell phone with your own money. It's a good sign that you are having some fun with your friends. We will continue to watch and listen and pray and hope that it keeps improving.

If it does, we will continue to help with college. No other conditions or deals are being put on you. We are not forcing you to see a therapist, although we strongly feel that would be beneficial, especially if you went in with the right attitude and mindset. We are not making you see a nutritionist. We are not making you weigh in or insist on certain weights by certain dates. We are not forcing you to stop over-exercising. You need to do what you deem necessary to get well. That is the only way it will work anyway. Give us a bill from Albion from this term. Then we will cut you checks periodically with no set schedule, as long as we feel like we are being treated with respect, you are not isolating yourself from the world, and you are gaining weight to feel better, look better, and get stronger.

This is a conditional promise. You have told me for over a year that if we paid for college, you would have no problem putting the weight on at all. You said that was the only thing holding you back from wanting to gain the weight back so . . . we'll see if you were being honest about that. We've seen you put twelve pounds on in just August. We've seen you put twenty pounds on in two months. So, I guess you do have a point. If you want to gain the weight, you can.

If no progress is seen, payments will not progress either. You can do it your way. If you do not put weight on, at least you'll know that you need help because all the excuses will be gone.

I love you more than you could possibly know, TJ. More than anything in the world, I hope and pray this will all work out.

Mom xo

9

If At First You Don't Succeed

IT WAS TJ's junior year of college and we were back to Square One. He was starting school looking way too thin. I was petrified to let him out of my sight, but absolutely helpless to do anything about it. I continued to try to engage him in conversation about his health, plead with him, make him see reason—but it had all been said before. At least TJ was more honest in his responses now.

"TJ, do you see yourself as too thin?" I asked him at one point.

"Mom, yes," he said. "If I could just gain muscle and not fat, I'd be happy to put weight on...."

"Remember the personal trainer we tried, and what she said?" I kept trying to reach him but I could see in his eyes that I wasn't getting through. Finally I just said what I was thinking: "Honey, why do you work so hard to look so bad?"

His response was this email:

I never said I am happy with the way I look. I look like crap. If I could snap my fingers and look like I did in my senior pictures, believe me, I would pay lots of money for that. I see puffy eyes, gray teeth, skeleton face. I hate that I can't stand how I look. But, the other part of that is I like so much the satisfaction I get from doing what I do or whatever; so they cancel each other out and I just stay where I am. You get confused with me being happy and me liking how I look. I hate how I look and I wish I looked better. But people have things that they don't like about themselves (you and your thin hair! Just kidding!) It doesn't mean I'm not happy though. I ask what people think about how I look because I just want to know what they think. I don't know how to put it. I'm curious. I ask questions. You know that. That is how I learn: asking questions.

There was a new restaurant TJ wanted to try so I took him there before he started back to school. The scene that unfolded was typical of our restaurant adventures. He didn't touch his wonton soup (said it was nasty). The waitress asked if he would like to try another kind and he politely said, "No thank you." I gobbled mine down. It was delicious. They brought his vegetables and rice but they were stir-fried, not steamed, and had some sauce on them. He wouldn't eat any. He didn't want any tea because it had caffeine in it, so he asked for a glass of water and then dumped two packets of NutraSweet into it. Of course he didn't eat the fortune cookie. So, all he ate was steamed rice.

We had given TJ $150 towards a cell phone for one of his Christmas presents. TJ and I spent half an hour in a cell phone store while he asked every question I could imagine about every phone, and finally picked one out. When it was time to purchase a calling plan, TJ said, "Mom, will you pay for a two-year plan as gifts for my next two birthdays?"

"TJ," I said, knowing that he had plenty of money

saved, "we gave you some money toward a phone. You need to pick up the rest of the cost yourself."

"Forget it then," he said, and started to walk out of the store.

"TJ! You really need to take some responsibility for part of this. You have money . . ."

"I won't spend my money because money is the one thing no one can take away from me," he said flatly—and walked out the door.

I hurried to keep up with him, throwing an apologetic look back at the nice young man who had waited on us for nearly an hour.

These maddening incidents only verified in my mind that TJ's illness was progressing. In an attempt to keep him safe, I wrote another letter to Albion but this time, instead of writing to the president, I wrote to the dean of students.

Dear Sir:

This is to inform you as to TJ's health concerns and our fear for his life and well-being. He was seen by Dr S. in the fall of 2004 and had very elevated liver enzymes. His AST (SCOT) was 69 (normal is 10–40). His ALT (SGPT) was 91 (normal is 2–45). Dr S informed me that TJ emphatically stated he was not to discuss any of his appointments with his mother Dr. S. went into counsel to find out if he could commit TJ. He called me with two phone numbers and said that I would have to do that and sounded quite desperate. He asked me, "Is TJ going in the hospital?" I told him that he needed to, but wouldn't go. I pleaded with TJ to go get help at a residential facility because he was looking worse. He looked as thin as he did when he blacked out and was in a car accident a year ago. He had a heart doctor appointment that he would not tell me about He carries around hand warmers and has layers of clothing on, even in the house, because his body temperature is so cold. He dumps packets upon packets of Equal in everything and on everything, even in his noodle soup (this is a common behavior—to use spices, sauces, and sugars that have 0 calories and 0 fat to give flavor to tasteless, fat-free food). He is still doing an hour of sit-ups in the morning and spends a couple of hours daily at the gym. He will not eat fat and only eats one time a day before going to bed at night. We are extremely concerned as he goes back to college this week. He will be in a single room alone and will be exercising fanatically in the weight room very early or late when few, if anybody will see him. He has not seen a therapist since last spring and we fear he is even better at hiding this illness. We very strongly feel he should be monitored at Albion by Dr. D., with weekly weigh-ins and monthly blood tests to ensure that he does not get worse. We also think he should not be allowed in the weight room unsupervised. TJ has promised us he will go to residential treatment in May, at the end of this term. We are just very concerned that we keep him safe until then. You may not feel you are legally obligated, but I feel you have a moral responsibility for the fact that TJ will spiral downhill without intervention.

Sincerely,

Susan Barry

In the middle of the first semester of his junior year, TJ told me he was not challenged enough on the Honors Business track and found his studies boring. He was having an increasingly difficult time deciding whether to stick with it—probably because he wasn't sure it was the *perfect* choice. He went to his counselor and took a test. She suggested to him that he might be well suited to the profession of dentistry, with his perfectionist personality and attention to detail.

He talked to me about it on his next trip home.

"Mom, I'll get a masters in business and have the top grade point in my class. But . . . do you think someone would actually hire me looking the way I do? I look like I'm 12 years old. On the other hand, have you ever heard of a dentist out of work? Maybe I could be a pediatric dentist. At least to kids, I'll look a little older!"

I understood what he was feeling and thinking; his argument made sense.

Once TJ had decided to change majors, he needed to enroll in extra classes to catch up—and for that, he had to get special permission. The college didn't ordinarily allow students to take three labs, but TJ talked them into making an exception so that he could take Organic Chemistry, Inorganic Chemistry and Biochemistry along with his other classes—an almost superhuman workload and the perfect excuse for isolating himself in his room 24/7. I never worried for a second that he couldn't do the work. TJ could do anything he put his mind to.

Except *eat*.

I knew my son. But as hard as I tried, I just couldn't understand how anyone who was starving himself and totally obsessed with thoughts of food, weight, calories, and exercise could possibly concentrate on schoolwork at all—let alone succeed in all of those challenging classes? During his second semester, TJ's weight started plummeting, most likely triggered by the stress of it all. Again, I pleaded with him to go to residential treatment.

"Honey, you know you left too early the first time. This time, you need to stay until *they* decide you are ready to go—and not leave when *you* decide it's time."

"Mom," he pleaded. "I'm only eight weeks from completing the hardest semester of my life! We paid the money and I put in all the time and everything! You just can't make me throw that away!"

We agreed he could finish the term if he promised to go to residential as soon as he was done and stay as long as they said he should. We had a deal—but for eight long, agonizing weeks, I couldn't sleep. Every time the phone rang, my heart stopped.

When spring finally arrived and the semester was winding down, something happened to interfere with the plan. TJ informed us that yes, he still intended to go back to residential, but on one condition. He hadn't done well enough in his Organic Chemistry class to ensure his acceptance into dental school. He insisted on retaking it while getting treatment. He understood that first, he'd need permission from Rogers, the treatment facility; and second, he'd have to find a class being offered during the summer.

I got my "I told you so's" out immediately: "TJ, there's a reason why the school didn't want you to take three labs at once! Plus, you promised you'd check into residential at the end of the term, no conditions! Honestly, at this point I don't care whether you get into dental school or not. What good is a degree if I have to place it in your coffin?"

I was so upset that I made him pretty upset, too. But of course he had an answer for everything.

"Mom, I had to take all of those classes to catch up to all of the other pre-med students! Remember, I was taking all business classes. I don't want to wait a whole other year because of one class! I have to retake that class this summer because I have to apply to dental schools this fall, before my senior year!"

The panic left my voice and I replied quietly. "Then you better find the class and make it happen. I really don't care if you start dental school in five years, TJ. Your health is much more important than anything else."

The team at Rogers gave the go-ahead for him take an on-line class while in residence. This was a great relief to me—I was sure that would be the toughest obstacle. I was wrong. TJ searched the entire country for an on-line Organic Chemistry class but, apparently, none existed. They all required lab attendance.

He called Michigan State, which is five minutes from our home, and begged. He got nowhere. He called again and this time managed to get through to the secretary of the professor who taught the class he wanted to take. TJ was very honest with her about his reason for wanting to take the class online, including the fact that he needed to get help with an eating disorder. He evidently won her heart: She agreed to talk to the professor.

After several more calls from TJ the following day, the secretary finally called him back with bad news. The professor had said absolutely not. He had no intention of posting lab notes on the Internet for one student. TJ should understand that this class was extremely challenging to pass even when attending every class in person.

This was not hard for me to believe. When I looked at TJ's Organic Chemistry notes, they looked like hieroglyphics or equations from another planet! Again, we argued about promises and priorities, goals and time-tables. TJ remained adamant.

"Mom, I want to live up to our deal but I will *not* go to Rogers unless I can take that class." In a quieter voice, he added, "You and I would never argue about anything if I didn't have this stupid problem, would we?"

He was right about that. I knew how lucky I was to have a son with exemplary moral values; who studied and worked harder than anyone; who saved his money; who appreciated everything we did for him; who never swore, drank or stayed out too late; who was clean, organized, dependable, honest, fun, athletic, creative—and even read the Bible. How could a mother argue with a kid like that? How could a kid like that starve himself?

TJ had everything going for him, including many people who respected, admired and loved him. He could motivate himself to accomplish just about anything—except for the one thing that was, for most people, the easiest thing in the world to do.

TJ was relentless about finding a class, continually searching the Internet and phoning several universities. He even called that poor secretary again. She must have been one of the many angels that followed TJ around during the eight and a half years he struggled with anorexia. Having taken his struggle to heart—believing that he was a sick kid trying to get well who deserved a break—she somehow convinced the professor to deviate from protocol and accept him as an online student.

She called TJ back and told him that the professor had very reluctantly agreed, but that TJ would have to study the textbook on his own, with no help from the professor. He would then be required to show up in person to take the 15-page final exam, the result of which would constitute his total grade. The professor warned that most students did poorly on the exam. He wanted to make it clear to TJ that it was highly unlikely that his grade would improve, as most students passed his class based on the sum of all of their work, not just their final exam grades.

TJ jumped at the offer. When I expressed my doubts about this plan, he insisted, "Don't worry, Mom, I can do it."

Armed with his textbook and his drive to succeed, off TJ went to residential treatment for the second time—and not a moment too soon. He looked horribly thin and pale, he was always freezing cold, and he had stopped laughing. His body seemed as if it were possessed by someone or something else.

I wanted my son back! I wanted to hear that contagious giggle again. I was relieved that he was going to be back in treatment, but when it was time to leave him at Rogers, I could barely let him go. Our hug was painful and sad, and we held each other for a long time as we both sobbed.

TJ's first stop was the in-patient hospital for two weeks, so that they could stabilize his condition and bring his weight up to a less dangerous spot. They pumped him full of whatever was necessary in order to begin to correct his body chemistry. According to TJ, they even had to order him a special mattress because he had a huge growth on his tailbone from doing so many sit-ups. They also put a brace on his leg because he had torn something or sprained his ankle (also from over-exercising), and something was wrong with his foot.

Because he was over 18, I really wasn't privy to what was going on with TJ—and this was a major frustration. In my opinion, the right to privacy should not apply in cases of anorexia, an illness in which hiding the truth is an actual symptom! I knew I couldn't trust my otherwise honest son when it came to the subjects of weight, food or exercise, so I was desperate for information from those in charge of his care. Besides that—can you think of any other illness where the patient doesn't *want* to get well?

TJ kept his promise and stayed the entire three months prescribed. He gained 37 pounds. At first he complained about everything, especially about all of the "weirdos" there. He did become very close friends with a young man named Daniel and considered the two of them to be the "cool guys." According to TJ, he and Daniel were the smart ones. They helped everyone else, talked sports constantly, and understood each other. They even helped each other eat by presenting each other with little challenges (Daniel's was eating bananas and TJ's was eating dessert). Together they laughed and played games to quench their thirst for competition, and when he wasn't with Daniel, TJ studied, studied, studied.

Eventually, he was reprimanded for the amount of time he was spending away from the group—but TJ insisted that his free time was *free* and that he should be permitted to spend it any way he wanted. Some patients chose napping, watching TV or putting puzzles together. He chose studying organic chemistry. In typical fashion, TJ rallied his fellow patients and asked for a meeting with the head of his unit. They all stood behind him in insisting that TJ was being discriminated against by the therapist, and that she should back off and leave him alone. As usual, TJ took control of the situation and got what he wanted.

*TJ made this mask during an art therapy session.
The front of it describes how TJ believes the world sees him.
The other side of the mask (behind the bars) shows what he
actually feels inside.*

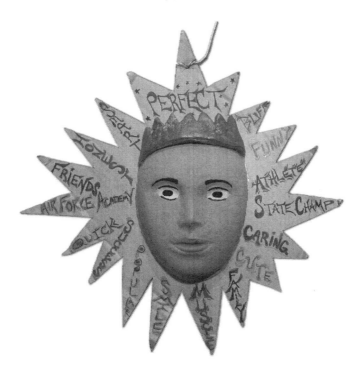

*Notice that the most prominent positive word
(above the crown) is "perfect."*

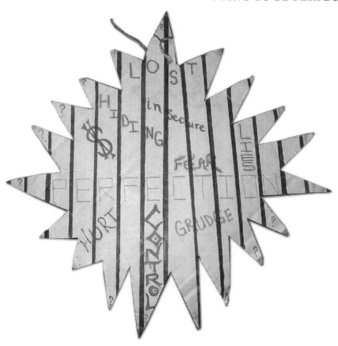

The most prominent negative word is "perfection."
Clearly, TJ understood that perfection can be a
double-edged sword—or two sides of the same mask.

Though he wasn't done with his treatment, TJ did fly back to East Lansing to take his final exam with classmates he'd never met and a professor he'd never heard. Rogers had given him a 24-hour pass. I dropped him off on campus, wished him good luck, and left. I wasn't sure who was more nervous or whose heart was pounding faster, his or mine. After returning to Rogers, TJ called the professor's secretary twice a day asking for news of his grade. When she finally had the information, she reported to TJ that the professor walked into the office, threw TJ's exam on her desk, and mumbled something about "that son-of-a-gun." He got the second-highest grade in the class!

Next came the much-feared DAT (Dental Admissions Test), for which he had been preparing at the same time he was studying organic chemistry. He had made arrangements to take it in Wisconsin, about an hour away from the treatment center, and once again he was given a day pass.

That experience was one of the most stressful TJ ever had to endure. My heart went out to him, as only a mother's could, as he told me the story. He was supposed to be picked up at 7 a.m. for a ride to the university where the test would be administered. TJ stood by the door waiting, with rising panic, until 7:20, when the car finally appeared. The driver assured him she would get him there on time, but nothing she promised could calm him down. Barely waiting for the car to come to a stop, TJ flew into the testing center and ran up to a table to register. To his horror, he was asked for two pieces of ID. He had none.

TJ's mind was racing. What excuse could he offer? Embarrassed as he was, he knew he had to tell the truth.

"Um . . . ," he began haltingly, "I am currently getting treatment for a . . . health issue at a hospital and I got a ride here and . . . I don't have my wallet."

Unmoved, the registrar informed him that without identification, he couldn't proceed; just as stubbornly, TJ insisted that he be permitted to take the test.

After two or three phone calls, a supervisor relented and TJ was told he could take it.

Phew.

"Do you think that I could please have five minutes to calm down before I start the exam?" he asked politely. "I am pretty upset now and I really need to stop shaking before I can even type my name!"

Five minutes later, he clicked the "begin" button on the computer.

When his time was up, TJ sat back in his chair waiting to receive his score. He told me later that he'd prayed harder at that moment than he'd ever done before and thought his heart was going to jump right out of his chest.

TJ passed every section with high scores. Guess which one he scored highest on? Organic Chemistry.

TJ's journal entry for that day said, "I passed the DAT today. I couldn't wait to call Dad and tell him my scores. I don't know if he was proud of me, though."

Not proud? That comment reminds me of something I read in a book about how an anorexic thinks. If someone were to say, "Hey, TJ, I really like that shirt you have on today!" he would think to himself, "Hmm, they didn't say they liked the shirt I had on yesterday. I must have looked terrible in it. I'm going to burn that shirt."

The first thing TJ wanted me to do after he told me the good news was to take chocolate chip cookies and flowers to the secretary who had helped him get into the chemistry class. He had already written her a thank-you letter. At the time, I shared TJ's boundless gratitude toward this woman; I believed she had saved his life! I only wished I were wealthy enough to buy her a trip instead of a bunch of flowers. I was used to feeling hopeless most of time, and the ray of light she provided did not go unappreciated.

Just as we had been the first time around, we were all afraid to have TJ come home from Rogers. It had felt so good to know he was safe and getting healthier by the day.

Following the protocol of the facility, TJ made a contract with his discharge team and therapists:

- I will make appointments with a therapist and a diet plan for the week that I discharge. I will also sign consents with all outpatient providers to communicate with one another as well as allow both parents to have monthly updates (more if necessary) to address any progress that I am making (i.e., maintaining weight) or any concerns that need to be addressed.
- I agree to follow up with an outpatient team and meet with a resident director and therapist at least one time a week until it is decided with my treatment team if it can be less often.
- I agree to be weighed at a minimum of one time a week at the Student Health Building. If my outpatient team would like more frequent weigh-ins, I will do so. I will also be weighed in shorts and a tee shirt.
- I agree to follow all recommendations of my outpatient treatment team, which includes exercise recommendations and meal plan increases.
- I agree to follow the established exercise regime and to only include more if it is recommended by my outpatient treatment team. If I feel I would like to include more, I will discuss it with my outpatient team.
- I agree to gain 2–3 pounds per week until I reach my goal weight of 120–125. If I am not gaining weight at this rate, I agree to increase my meal plan and follow it.
- I will continue working on open communication with my family, and before I leave, we will agree on a plan for "family activities" so that our relationships continue to progress.
- I will set aside Friday and Saturday night each week to "relax," take a study break, and do something fun.

- I will come to an agreement with my family regarding what food is and is not allowed in the house and we will deal with food and eating.
- I will complete my relapse prevention packet and present it before I leave.
- I will agree to seek a higher level of care if I do not continue to make progress of at least 2–3 pounds a week and not reach my goal weight. I also agree to withdraw from school if my weight goes below 110 for two consecutive weeks.

I UNDERSTAND THAT FAILURE TO FOLLOW ANY OF THE ABOVE IS NONCOMPLIANCE FROM TREATMENT AND MAY RESULT IN WITHDRAWING FROM SCHOOL.

TJ Warschefsky
08/11/05

In spite of the contract and TJ's much-improved appearance, it wasn't long before I was fighting the old battles. The very first morning he was home, he wanted fat-free cereal with skim milk for breakfast and he wanted to resume working out. He also wanted to come with me when I went grocery shopping so that he could control the type of food I bought.

I had been hoping with all my heart that TJ could finally sit at the kitchen table and be happy with whatever I served for dinner, but that wasn't the case—not even close. And he certainly didn't want us watching his every move.

"Why do you have to act like the food police all the time?" he yelled at us one night that first week. "When will you get it through your heads that I just spent the entire summer getting well? When will you *trust* me?"

Of course I would have loved to trust him, but I just didn't see the behavioral changes I'd been praying for.

TJ's senior year was looming. Soon he would be back in his single dorm room, studying and applying to dental schools. On one of our walks, in a lovely moment of honesty and closeness, he asked me if I believed he could stay well.

"TJ, why don't you answer that first?" I replied.

"No, Mom," he said. "You go first—but I promise to tell you what I really think afterwards."

I thought carefully and said, "I think that if you get into dental school, you'll be fine. If you don't, I'll be worried."

"Mom, I totally agree," he said.

I appreciated his clarity, but his answer didn't exactly make me feel sanguine about his future. Nobody's life is perfect. Disappointments are inevitable. Would we always have to worry about the next trigger?

10

Dr. Warschefsky

"MOM, DO YOU think I should have my patients just call me Dr. TJ? Hardly anybody can pronounce or spell *Warschefsky.*"

TJ's senior year of college was an exciting time for all of us, but a stressful time, too, because he was living alone, applying to dental schools, and continuing to struggle with his eating disorder.

TJ's routine hadn't changed much. He still wouldn't eat any fat and only ate at all between 8 p.m. and 10 p.m. During those two hours, he rewarded himself for completing his goals for that day. If he had attended all of his classes, done all of his homework, and exercised for four hours, he considered himself worthy of eating, answering his email, and watching "SportsCenter." He continued to come home every other weekend to do his laundry and we always took our walks, ate our ice cream, and talked about whatever he wanted to bring up.

He was doing well in all of his pre-med classes and was right on target for graduating in four years, despite the breaks he'd been forced to take while hospitalized or in residential treatment. He would have his Bachelors degree in economics and management with a concentration in public policy and professional management and a minor in cellular and molecular biology.

TJ waited anxiously for his mail every day, hoping to be granted an interview. He was well aware that many students don't make it into dental school right out of college and that the average age of acceptance is 24 (TJ was 21)—but that didn't discourage the future Dr. TJ!

When he came home at Christmas, I was worried, as usual, about how the family would react to his physical appearance at our holiday get-togethers. He could hide his rail-thin body under layers of winter clothes, but he couldn't hide his gaunt, chalk-white face. At this point, he really didn't look like himself. Because of his sunken cheeks, his teeth stuck out. So did his small ears. His eyes had no sparkle. There was downy hair all over him that I learned was called "lanugo." (This is a classic anorexia symptom—part of the body's desperate effort to stay warm.) His usual crown of thick, shiny hair had become dull and thin. The skin on his face was pulled tight over his bones, which protruded everywhere.

Another thing he couldn't hide from his aunts, uncles, cousins, and grandparents was how little he ate. At Christmas, most of us tend to splurge a little—but all anyone heard from TJ was an incessant, "No, thank you, I'm good." I knew how stressful it was for him when everyone sat down to eat. Well-meaning aunts and uncles would push food at him.

"Try this, TJ, it's good."

"I made this especially for you, TJ. You have to try it!"

"Come on, TJ, have just a few bites—it's delicious!"

I understood completely the frustration they felt; multiply it by a million and that would reflect my own frustration in dealing with TJ's issues for eight long years.

After the holidays, there were usually a few brave souls who would say something about how TJ looked or point out the fact that he didn't eat much. Someone would offer to talk to him or suggest things I could say. I wanted to scream, "*Nothing will work!*" But, I didn't ... partly out of politeness but mostly because I didn't want to believe it.

Not long after the holidays, the much-anticipated dental school letters started arriving. To keep track of everything, TJ took a sheet of paper and made three columns: The first was for the name of the dental school; the second was headed, "No, we cannot offer you a position at this time"; and the third said, "Yes, we would like to set up an interview." He posted it on the wall of his dorm room. Whenever a letter arrived, TJ would rip it open immediately and put an X in the appropriate place on his chart. He'd applied to about 15 schools, and the "no" column began to pull ahead fast.

With every "no," my heart sank with his. Thankfully, when all of the replies were in, he had three X's in the "yes" column—plenty—and we were both ecstatic. He was accepted at University of Michigan, Marquette and University of Detroit. I wondered if these three dental schools realized they were helping to save my son's life.

After visiting all three schools, he was most excited about Marquette University's program, and so was I. Among other things, the school is located in Milwaukee, just 30 minutes from Rogers Residential Hospital, which seemed like another miracle to me. If he were accepted there, it would be easy for TJ to continue to get support from Rogers.

He came back from his Marquette interview very excited, explaining that it was the newest dental school in the country. The lab provided each student with a "head" to work on and he couldn't stop talking about all of the "cool stuff" they had.

"Mom, I think I connected well with the dean who interviewed me," he bubbled. "Some big, tall dude came out of his interview right before me. When I went in, I said, 'Whoa, I think you need more short people around here!' Mom, the guy who interviewed me was about my height! He got a big kick out of that comment."

"That's great, honey," I said, beaming at my glimpse of the happy TJ who had gone into hiding lately. "Oh, my gosh, I am so proud of you."

Then came more waiting.

I honestly think one of the happiest days of my life was when TJ called me—surprisingly calm and collected—to tell me that he had been accepted to Marquette Dental School. I couldn't believe that yet another miracle had been granted to my son! Not only that, but he was also accepted to the two other schools at which he had interviewed. Surely now he would realize how much he had to live for, what a bright future lay ahead of him. Surely this would help him beat his insidious illness for good.

My son was the only student in his class to get into dental school. Because TJ felt sorry for all those who didn't make it, he started a "dental club" and made himself the first "guest speaker," in order to offer the others his advice on how to get in next time. He walked them through each of the steps he took in the hope that it would help them on their next try.

Dental school cost $56,000 a year and you already know TJ's views on spending money. He decided to apply to the Navy, Air Force and Army to see if he could get a medical scholarship that would cover all of his expenses, with the understanding that he would then serve as a military dentist for four years. It sounded like a great idea; little did we know how the endeavor would imperil TJ's life.

After he sent off his applications, the anxious waiting game began again. Ultimately, TJ was accepted into all three military branches—and in fact they seemed to be competing for him, which made him very happy. After doing some research, asking questions, and pondering his options obsessively, he decided to go with the Air Force.

TJ was required to attend Air Force boot camp for six weeks, either before or after dental school. Having previously enjoyed a summer at a leadership camp, he decided to go to boot camp before beginning dental school—though I strongly discouraged him because of his fragile physical condition. One look at his upper arms might jeopardize his scholarship!

He brushed my concerns aside with, "Oh, Mom, you're being such a *mom*. Stop worrying about me!"

"Ok, TJ, do what you want to do," I replied quietly. "But these guys are smart. They'll take one look at you and wonder what is going on with your health. They are bound to be very concerned with health issues because they are investing a lot of money in you and will want to make sure they're going to have a top-notch doctor at their disposal in a few years. I've heard that they won't even take someone with a peanut allergy!"

"Mom. Can't you see that now is the best time for me to get boot camp out of the way? I've got nothing to do all summer anyway. Once I graduate, I'll be eager to start my career!"

"Please, TJ," I begged. "I know you don't want to hear this, but I really wish you'd go back to residential one last time before school starts. You could stay three months without missing anything and then start school feeling really strong and healthy."

As usual, TJ was persuasive, if not completely right. "Mom, why would I go back a third time? If it hasn't helped by now, what could it change? It would be a waste of time! I know exactly what I need to know. I could run the therapy groups. I have all the dieticians' information memorized! They are not going to tell me one thing I don't already know and haven't heard a hundred times already. It's pointless!"

I tried one last tactic: "TJ, have you ever heard the saying, 'three's a charm'? Or... how about, 'if at first you don't succeed, try, try again'? You have everything going for you right now *except your health*. And if you don't have that, trust me, nothing else will matter!"

We debated until we were both tired and turned in without resolving anything. The next morning, TJ— always a loving son—said to me, "Mom, why don't we compromise? I'll go to boot camp and get it over with, and when I get back, I'll go back to residential for a 'tune-up' before I go to Marquette."

We both knew that plan would leave only a month for treatment—not long enough. I suspected that behind this plan was his desire to spend a month with Daniel, his best friend, who was at Rogers for the fourth time. When we talked about it, he confessed that he did have Daniel on his mind.

"But, Mom, I'm a little worried about how Daniel will feel if he sees me back at Rogers for the third time. Maybe it will make him feel hopeless ... like ... 'If TJ can't beat this disease, then nobody can.'"

"You know what, honey?" I said. "I think seeing you will make Daniel proud—because he'll see that you are being honest with yourself, admitting that you need help again, and being courageous enough to get it."

What I didn't say was that I figured TJ had been hiding the truth about his current condition from Daniel and didn't want to be found out.

As usual, TJ got his way and went off to boot camp. After two weeks, his superior officer called him in for a meeting and told him he was being sent home because he was "anemic." The official letter TJ received, which we didn't see until much later, revealed a different story. It listed the reason for his discharge as "Substandard Weight and Possible Eating Disorder."

TJ was thunderstruck.

"Why can't I just take iron pills?" he asked. "Sir, I've kept up with you on every single morning run. I came in second place out of everyone doing pull-ups. . . ." But this time TJ could not get his way. He was devastated. He knew he would now be responsible for paying for dental school. He lost his rank of Second Lieutenant and his Medical Service Corps full-ride scholarship to dental school.

In a frantic attempt to be reinstated into the Air Force, TJ summoned up all of his powers of persuasion and wrote this letter:

In the process of applying for the Air Force Health Professionals Scholarship Program, I was informed and assured that there was no minimum weight standard. I successfully completed the fitness and physical health examination that is required to enter into the armed services. In fact, I also applied to, and was accepted into, the Army and Navy branches of the HPSP as well. The Air Force assured me that my low weight would not in any way, shape, or form affect my status or participation in the program. I have been short with a small build for my entire life. My blood work was perfect and my physical conditioning was excellent.

While at CPT this past summer, I was in the top of my class (06–05) in all of the fitness testing and athletic events. I was chosen to represent my squadron in the pull-up challenge and the long-distance running events (I ran cross-country in college). My fitness scores were the best among my other flight members. I had absolutely no difficulty with the fitness regimen and actually felt as though I was not getting challenged enough in regards to my fitness and exercise; so I went to the workout facilities before or after programming. There was absolutely no questioning about my eating or anything regarding my health status—until I was weighed.

The circumstances concerning the weigh-in were confusing and unfortunate. The initial weigh-in process was very disorganized and disorderly; trying to get all of us CPT students in and out as quickly as possible. As I waited in line, I noticed major discrepancies in all of the tests that were being administered. Some were being weighed in shorts and tee shirts while others were wearing their camouflage gear and boots. I was one that was dressed in my full camouflage outfit with heavy boots. In addition, I had come directly from lunch (where we were instructed to drink four glasses of water). Needless to say my weight increased to a solid eight to nine pounds above the weight I know is normal for me.

Unfortunately, my normal weight was so low to begin with that even with the fluid, food, outfit, and boots it still caught the attention of the medical personnel. I was called in for a supplemental weigh-in, which was to be administered at 0600. I was the only person there and I was weighed in shorts and shirt, prior to eating and drinking. Not surprisingly my weight was significantly less than the initial reading. Although I had been performing at the top of my class in the physical fitness activities and I had been previously informed that the weight is a non-issue, I knew these results would be looked into.

The apparent drastic drop in weight obviously set off red flags, and I was subjected to three days of intense blood work CAT scans, EKGs, echocardiograms, and every other test that could possibly explain the weight loss. I had to miss significant class time and was treated differently from the rest of the COT students. I was not allowed to participate in the PT each morning and I could not even march in line with my flight. I felt isolated and betrayed, without just reason or cause. Every single test came back with the same result: I was in perfect health. The sole exception was that my blood work revealed slight anemia. Anemia is a condition that can be easily fixed with a pill or an increased consumption of certain nutrients, and I was given pills to rectify this deficiency. However, my case was further reviewed by internists and doctors throughout the Air Force. All of the tests indicated that I was systematically healthy so I was labeled as a possible eating disorder candidate.

I will openly admit that I was not eating very much in the cafeteria. I was certainly not prepared for the strict and regimented dining room atmosphere. Additionally, the intense heat surely left me dehydrated since I typically do not drink very much. I have been told my entire life that I live a military style life. I love the discipline, organization and strict regime of the Air Force. However, I was just caught off guard when I discovered we had a set, short amount of time to eat, were not allowed to speak, and had to chug down four glasses of fluids. The first few days I bought a lot of food and drinks and was only able to finish a very small portion of it because of the time and fluid restrictions. I am extremely careful and vigilant with my money and the thought of wasting all that food was very bothersome to me. In response, I decided to eat less at mealtime, and to buy groceries for eating in my room. This allowed me to eat a small amount in the dining hall and not feel rushed, as well as not feel guilty about wasting food and money. Due to the results of the weigh-in, I was also put on watch at the cafeteria for a couple of days. However, I had purchased all those groceries and was already eating in my room. Not wanting the food I had purchased to go to waste, I would still eat very little in the cafeteria.

I was both heartbroken and disappointed to learn that the Air Force had decided that a "substandard weight and possible eating disorder" were disqualifying me from the program. I had done everything that was asked of me and was subjected to a battery of tests which I had passed with flying colors. In fact, Colonel M [the director of the program] sat me in his office and promised me that my early departure from COT would not affect my status in the Air Force. I feel very strongly that the actions may have been taken prematurely and without proper consideration. I have not been contacted for any explanations, directions, or questions about this situation. I would appreciate the chance to better explain the situation if the committee still feels as though a disqualification is warranted. There is only so much I can write on this sheet of paper without writing a book or not answering any other questions that may still lurk. I do not want to inundate the committee with information that is already known or is perhaps irrelevant.

After being informed that I would have to leave COT because of my slightly anemic condition and "possible eating disorder," I immediately addressed the issues that they felt hindered my ability to serve in the Air Force. There is nothing more that I want to do than to be an Air Force dentist, so I was and still am willing to follow any orders that would enhance my participation in the program. I am no longer anemic. I sought out counseling for my "possible" eating disorder, and was able to put on weight. I have had difficulty putting on weight in the past, and have previously been referred to dieticians and therapists to help with this situation in which I have successfully gained weight without any feelings of remorse, guilt or hesitation. My daily activity level and schedule are very intense and my metabolism is extremely high so I need to monitor my weight more closely than most do to ensure that my weight stays up. As mentioned, my physical conditioning is excellent, and I would love the opportunity to prove this with any physical examinations that are deemed necessary in order for my reinstatement If, after reading this explanation, the committee still feels that I should be disqualified, I would appreciate it if I could be contacted to elucidate any misunderstandings. I belong in the Air Force and would like the opportunity to clarify any discrepancies.

A career in dentistry and the ability to serve my country are two goals that I have had for as long as I can remember I am on my way to becoming a competent dentist and my only request is to know what it will take for me to be back on track serving in the Air Force. I strongly feel as though this relationship is mutually beneficial. I strongly desire to become a medical professional in the Air Force; and I can promise that the Air Force will appreciate and benefit from my talents and contributions. I am overly eager and completely enthusiastic about every single aspect of being an Air Force dentist for life. I am fully aware that the HPSP and the armed forces in general are lacking resources in regards to medical professionals such as what I will become.

Please contact me, at your convenience, with any questions or further information that you desire.

The letter was written on January 27, 2007, two weeks before TJ died.

TJ did keep his promise to get treatment after boot camp and off he went to Rogers. This time, he had offered to take the boat from Muskegon to Milwaukee, where someone from the residential facility could pick him up.

I'll never forget leaving him at that boat station. I couldn't believe he actually agreed to go a third time. I so hoped that this visit would be enough to take that insidious, impossible, horrific illness from him. I sensed that he was genuinely trying to get well, *wanting* to get well. I don't know what I would have done in a similar situation. Understanding what an act of strength and bravery it was for him to get on that boat alone and go to a place he hated, my heart bled for him. But did he really hate it there? Maybe he felt normal there. Maybe he felt safe and well there. Maybe he anticipated his stay at Rogers as a relief from the stress and pressure of living in a world where nobody understood him.

It was hard for me to guess what he was feeling—but when we hugged, his eyes filled with tears and he whispered in my ear, "I don't want to go, Mom."

He went.

When I arrived to pick him up a month later, against the recommendation of Rogers but at TJ's insistence, TJ met me at the door. I was shocked at the sight of him, still gaunt and hollow-eyed. Daniel took me aside and said that he was very concerned that TJ wasn't ready to leave yet—and of course he was right.

Later, after TJ had passed away, I received his records from Rogers. The notes of the doctors and nurses made it clear that he hadn't made much progress during that visit. He had been noncompliant at meals and refused to challenge himself. He had re-entered Rogers on July 10, 2006, at a weight of 84.4 pounds and was released on August 11, 2006, at 89.8 pounds. He was 21 years old.

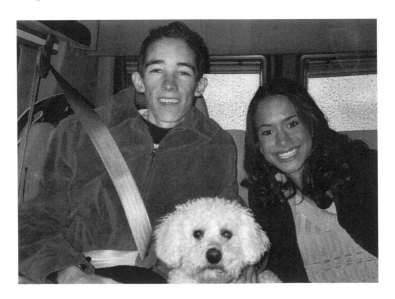

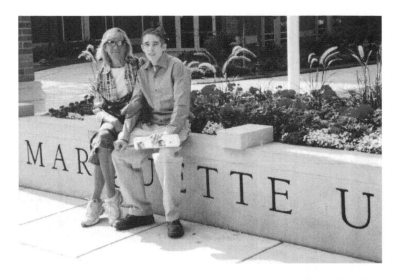

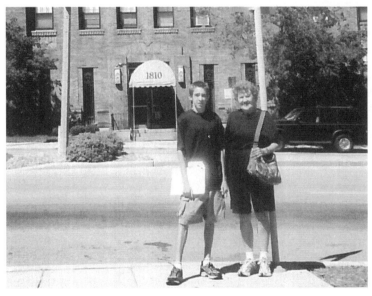

Little did we imagine, he would die in his new apartment that he was so proud to show his grandma.

11

Marquette Bound!

ON ONE OF our last walks, just before TJ went off to dental school, he expressed the changes he wanted to make in his behavior.

"First of all, Mom, I want to make life-long friends," he said, as we strolled along and ate our ice cream. "I realize that at Albion, I isolated myself too much. I mean, I barely had any friends other than Phyllis in the kitchen!"

I didn't say anything at that moment, but I remember being glad he said that. When I had visited him at Albion, no one had ever walked by us and said, "Hey, TJ!" It made me sad at the time, because he'd been so popular in elementary, middle and high school.

This disease systematically robs you of your friends, relatives and social life. And then it goes after your *life*.

The next thing TJ said to me on that walk was not something I wanted to hear.

"Mom," he said firmly, "I'm afraid I'll never make it being so far from you."

"Yes, you will, honey," I insisted. "Remember, we'll always be underneath the same big sky. And every time you hear a mourning dove sing hoo-hoo-hoo, pretend it's me saying 'I-love-you.' " I tried to sound convincing as I slung my arm over his bony shoulders. Now I just had to convince *myself*.

TJ and I drove to Milwaukee one weekend to find him an apartment. It was an absolutely unbelievable experience. From TJ's computer in Okemos, Michigan, he planned and arranged for us to visit 10 apartment complexes in one afternoon. He made all the appointments and marked up a map and off we started on foot. Our appointments were spaced efficiently throughout the afternoon—the first at 1 p.m., the next at 1:30, and so on. He'd planned everything so expertly that we arrived for each viewing at exactly the appointed time, often to find the apartment manager waiting for us outside.

Ten appointments, 10 apartments, 10 managers, all in one afternoon. I flashed back to high school and TJ's pool parties. If we'd asked that he end a party at 10 p.m., he somehow got 30 teenagers to clean up, thank us and walk out the front door just as our mantel clock was striking 10 chimes. At the time, I marveled at his organizational skills, but by the time of our apartment-hunting adventure, I couldn't help but see this behavior as obsessive compulsive—and a symptom of much deeper problems. In the end, TJ wound up in an apartment right across from the dental school—the cheapest one we looked at!

Striving to be perfect can be a wonderful thing. Dying to be perfect is not.

TJ's dental school schedule stretched from 8 a.m. to 5 p.m. every day. He was taking 24 credits and he loved it!

He called me one day, all excited: "Hey Mom, I got voted treasurer of the dental club! I think it was because of my speech. I told them I know I'm short, but I have never been short of money. That's mostly because I'm the cheapest person you'll ever meet. I'm hardworking, meticulous in record keeping, very organized, and love to save money! I even wear socks that have holes in them … and then I took off my shoe and showed them! By the time I was done, the whole class was laughing. Then the other guy got up to give his speech and said, 'Ok, I'm going to tell you right now, I can't compete with that!'"

TJ held a fundraiser for the school, coming up with all kinds of creative ideas and making a tidy sum of money for its treasury.

When he died at age 22, he had $56,000 in his savings account. He had saved all of his birthday, Christmas and lawn-cutting money, plus every dime he'd made working for his dad. Ironically, that was just about exactly the cost of one year of tuition.

I believe TJ never considered the possibility that he could really die from his illness. After he was gone, we learned that he could have had a $100,000 life insurance policy that was free to the Marquette dental students. All he had to do was fill out a form. He never bothered.

The next semester—TJ's last on this earth—he again took 24 credits, standard for the program. I really couldn't imagine how he and his classmates could study, concentrate and memorize so much information. And of course, in his case, this was while his mind was filled with thoughts of food, calories, weight, and exercise.

Research indicates that the brain is the very last organ to succumb to this disease. Our instinct for survival—for nourishment—is the final thing to go, even if we resist answering its call.

I want to say a little more about the disease itself, so I'm going to move away from TJ's story and tell you about something that happened to a family I met in a support group I started after we lost TJ.

The group was intended for families of patients, not the patients themselves, because I knew I couldn't really help them. My purpose was to create a safe place where parents, siblings and friends of anorexics could come together, gain a better understanding of the illness, and share their thoughts, feelings and coping strategies.

For a family, dealing with an eating disorder is one of the most difficult and emotionally draining challenges there is. Why? Because it is so hard for anyone to understand that anorexic behavior isn't a choice.

As a family member or friend of an anorexic, we start out in denial that there's a real problem. This evolves into sympathy—but then comes anger. There's a cure right in the kitchen! Why won't he or she take it? We plead and reason and talk until we're blue in the face, but nothing gets through.

I wanted these frustrated families and friends to know they weren't alone—that others were experiencing the same frustration and pain. That is why I began the group.

One evening, without warning me, a mom and dad brought their daughter who was struggling with severe anorexia to our meeting. I didn't want to turn them away, of course, but I tabled what I had intended to discuss and decided to talk about TJ instead. I guess I was hoping to shock this young girl a little bit—to make her see that imminent death was a real possibility for her, not just something that happened to other people.

After sharing some memories of my son, I read a very moving poem that he had written while in treatment.

Yo Quiero

I've cried, I've lied, I've nearly died;
I've sinned, I've binged, I've felt so pinned;
I've not eaten, I've lost weight, I ruined my fate;
I've obsessed, had no rest, but always aced the test.
For the longest time I would insist that there was nothing
     wrong,
I was living my life in my own desire, and dancing to my
     own song.
The doctors and therapists, the experts and counselors,
just never had the answer,
It was like I contracted an awful disease, much similar to
     cancer.
My family cried, because they tried, to help and be my
     guide;
They tried control, they tried patrol, they tried to save my
     soul;
I ignored the clues, I had a short fuse, and so much did I
     lose;
I chose not to see, its power on me, and for this I paid a
     large fee.
Like I had done for so many years, I was lured into a trap,
Although they were just trying to help—they were
     through with all my crap.
I hated the stay but realized how close I came to dying,
But was so enraged from all I had missed, that I just
stopped my trying.
All the years, and all the tears, and all the scary fears;
My lying, my crying, my false claims to trying;
Through all of the pain, the runs in the rain, what little did
     I gain;
I finally confessed, this was far from the best, I badly
     needed a rest.

Although I dissented to me getting help,
in my head I recognized need,
My life was in overdrive and I could not handle the
overwhelming increasing speed.
I went to groups, I went to meals, I even had my snack,
And quickly I learned my desire to change,
was the only thing holding me back.
I remembered the fears and many tears from over all the
    years,
Who I kissed and what I missed, and how often I was
    pissed;
At times I was well, and it was so clear to tell,
I was free from my little cell;
But when I was bad, I lost all I had, and always felt very
    mad.
I surrendered myself and made a big pact,
that this time *I want* to get healthy,
So I can enjoy my life, my college, my friends,
the possibilities are so very wealthy.
I realized how much I had lost, and decided it was
    enough,
I have so much going that there is no need to make my life
    so rough.
I want to be strong, to do no more wrong, and to live a life
    so long;
All it took was desire, to step out of the fire, and a new life
    to acquire;
It was nothing I lack, that was holding me back,
my thoughts were just out of whack;
It's like I took a pill, that gave me the will, to finally see
    over the hill.
I can't wait to get home, step out of my dome,
and start my brand new poem.

Understandably, I could barely get through the poem, but somehow I made it to the end. By then, everyone's eyes were filled with tears and no one spoke for a few long moments. When I couldn't bear the silence any longer, I turned to the young girl and asked, "Could you relate to any of what TJ wrote?"

I don't think anyone who was in that room will soon forget her answer.

"Oh, my gosh, yes, almost all of it," she began. "But, to tell you the truth . . . the whole time you were reading it, I was throwing up little bits in my mouth. I was thinking about how mad I was that my lunch plan had gotten changed. I was only going to have a little yogurt, but instead my dad wanted to have lunch with me, so I had a huge salad. When I got home, my stomach was so bloated and big, I was disgusted with myself. I wanted to take the kitchen butcher knife and just cut my stomach off!"

I couldn't have come up with a more eloquent example of how the anorexic mind works. This poor girl may have heard TJ's words, but she didn't hear the meaning. She was trapped inside her own obsession and her parents—all of us—were on the outside looking in.

TJ worked hard at dental school. We talked and emailed daily and he honestly sounded good on the phone: happy, busy and motivated to do well. When Thanksgiving week came around, he told me he was too busy studying to come home, but that he was going to make himself a big Thanksgiving dinner and eat it.

Sure you are, TJ, I thought.

A few days later, he sent me "proof"—pictures he had

taken of all the food he'd made. I suppose you could call it a feast, although the entire meal had been modified to be fat free.

As Christmas got closer, we started making plans for me to pick him up. TJ loved Christmas. He talked me into spending five days with him in Milwaukee, doing some fun things he intended to plan, before we headed home. I didn't realize it at the time, but the real reason he wanted me there for five days was so that we could spend time together before he broke the news that he wasn't planning to come home at all. He knew how horrible he looked at that point; he knew how upset the family would be if they saw him.

When I arrived at his apartment, he immediately took me over to the dental lab to show me his cubicle and the mannequin head that he practiced on. On the way out, we ran into the dean who had helped make TJ's dream of dental school come true. I shook hands with him and we wished each other a Merry Christmas. Just before we parted, he looked me straight in the eye and said, "Please take good care of our TJ, Mrs. Barry."

I knew what he meant. "I'm trying my absolute best," I said. The look we exchanged spoke louder than our words. It was full of concern and fear.

12

The Best and Worst of Times: My Last Visit

STILL THINKING THAT TJ and I would be going home at the end of our Milwaukee adventure, I was excited about all of the fun things he had on our agenda. Being the consummate planner, he'd figured out how to schedule our activities around his class schedule and other commitments—but one day, he apologized for not being able to spend a lot of time with me. He had signed up to go to an elementary school and give free teeth cleaning and checkups.

He returned very excited. He'd been in the restroom when some of the second graders came in and had overheard one of them whisper, "Hey, you guys! One of the dentists is in here!" TJ was so proud to be admired. "See, Mom," he said. "I think I really should consider being a pediatric dentist. At least I would look tall and grown up to *them*!"

I smiled and agreed he would be awesome at that. Kids had always liked TJ and the feeling was mutual.

The next day, we went to the Milwaukee Art Museum, but TJ seemed preoccupied. He was second-guessing himself again.

"Mom, I don't know if I made the right decision about this dental school thing."

"What are you talking about, TJ?" I asked, dumbfounded.

"I think of some of my buddies who finished college and got regular nine-to-five jobs making $50,000 a year. They have lots more time to play sports, go to games, have fun . . . meanwhile, I'm *paying* $56,000 a year to go to dental school! It kills me to think what my debt will be after four years! Do you really think it's worth it?"

That was TJ: frugal to a fault. "Honey, you will pay that back in no time!" I said. "All doctors and dentists have debt. You have to think long-term. You'll pay it all back and you'll be making enough money to go to any game you want! As a dentist, you could even schedule three-day weekends!"

"But what do I need all that money for, Mom? You know one of my problems is I can't spend it anyway."

Poor TJ, overthinking things, trapped in his obsessions and in his mind's own vicious cycle. I felt terrible for him. He was right about the money, of course. He had trained himself to live on very little and had a difficult time spending anything he had. I knew this was related to his eating disorder—it was just another version of self-denial and self-control.

Was it about security? For a long time, he had hoarded money, gum, food, everything he owned. He wouldn't open up a new pair of socks until the pair he was wearing was full of holes. Did he think he was unworthy of having new things?

I later worked with the family of an anorexic 26-year-old. They told me that their daughter declined spending two dollars out of every paycheck to have health insurance.

After TJ was done with his classes the next day, he took me on a more detailed tour of his school. He was so proud to show me his lab coat with his name embroidered on it. As we went around the lab, he told me about each of his 79 fellow students, where they were from, and something about each one. He lit up as he talked about his friends, telling me how nice they all were, how ridiculously smart they were, how he talked sports constantly with this one and so admired another's character. I thought how unusual it was for someone his age to have nothing but positive feelings for a group of students from such varied backgrounds.

"I'm hearing nothing but good things about all of them, TJ! Aren't there any 'weirdos' in this whole room of 80?"

"Mom, not a one," he said.

I sat through 79 pictures and 79 mini-stories, so happy that he was happy.

That night, he took me to a neighborhood that was well known for its enormous display of Christmas lights. He knew I would love it and I did. The night after that, he took me to a Marquette basketball game—his highlight of the week. It was great to see him excited and happy, but for me, the way TJ looked cast a shadow over the festivities. He was so thin, so pale, so cold, and severely lacking in energy. He told me that sometimes, when he was walking with his friends, he had to pretend to have to go to the bathroom because he couldn't keep up with them.

I could not believe my ears. This wasn't the same TJ who had been nicknamed "quick as a cat" by his tennis friends. I told him for the millionth time that he needed "fuel to run the car," food to have energy, strength, and good health … but I knew my words were not registering.

One thing that did make me happy was hearing many of the students who passed us yell, "Hey, TJ!" or "Teej!" TJ had fulfilled his vow to make dental school different from his four-year undergraduate experience, where he had "hidden out." At Marquette, he worked hard to make life-long friends, and after only four months, he'd made a good start. TJ could always accomplish any goal he set for himself.

The weekend arrived and we had it entirely to ourselves. On Sunday, we decided to go Christmas shopping since he hadn't bought any gifts yet. Afterward, we would go out to dinner and see a movie.

That night, I had to face the fact that TJ's state of mind was deteriorating—and it petrified me. His inability to make decisions and his obsessive-compulsiveness about time and schedules were glaring. TJ was more "TJ" than ever.

We went to the mall so that I could help him choose Christmas gifts. We shopped and shopped and he bought nothing. I got frustrated after a while and asked why he didn't like anything I suggested. He said he was just looking for ideas and that he had plenty of time to shop when he got home. I knew that behind his hesitancy was the fact that we were in nice department stores, not Wal-Mart or Meijer, where the prices would be lower.

"Mom, what show do you want to see?" he asked me, trying to deflect my attention from his empty shopping basket.

"You pick, honey," I said. "You don't get to go to the movies very often."

"No, Mom, I want you to enjoy it, so you pick."

We narrowed it down to three films we both wanted to see and I suggested that we each eliminate one. But even after I'd crossed one off the list, he refused to decide. "Just pick one, Mom. I'd like to see both of those."

I sighed and chose one.

"Now which theater do you want to go to?" he asked.

"Well, let's not decide that right now. We can figure it out after we're done with shopping and dinner, and we'll see what time it's getting to be, OK?"

His reply stung. "Mom, please don't do that to me. You know I have to have it all planned out."

I stopped looking through the racks and stared at him. He went into planning mode: "OK, the first show is about a mile and a half from here, but it's in the opposite direction from my apartment. Those show times are at 4:30, 6:20, 8:10, and 10. The second theater is two and a quarter miles from here, but it's on the way to my apartment. Those show times are 5, 6:50, 8:45, and 10:30."

I stood there speechless. He'd memorized all of it. "Well," I answered, "I picked the movie, so you pick the theater and time. Do you want to eat first?"

"I'm done shopping," TJ said casually. (He'd been done before we started.) "So maybe we should just go to the movie now. I think I'd rather eat after the movie anyway—so you pick the show time."

After the movie, which we both enjoyed, I said I was starving and asked where he wanted to eat. Again, we went through the "you choose, no you choose" dance.

"TJ, I picked what movie, what theater, what time. I will eat anywhere and anything. You know I am not the one with an eating problem, so you pick the restaurant." It was incredible to me that he could not choose even that.

By this time we were pulling out of the parking lot. "Just go anywhere, Mom. I will be able to eat something no matter what restaurant it is," he insisted. So I spun into a small diner that looked safe enough.

When the waitress asked if we were ready to order, TJ said we needed a few more minutes. I could tell he was getting anxious because he saw nothing on the menu that was fat free, sugar free or calorie free. For seven of the years TJ had been ill, he'd been concerned mainly with fat content. Recently, that had expanded to include sugar and calories. He'd consume none of them if he could help it. Along with his 24 credits and four hours of exercise, this contributed to a dangerous regimen, to say the least.

The waitress returned and when she asked TJ what he wanted, he turned to me and—as always—said, "Mom, why don't you order first?"

As I often did, I ordered much more food (all of it loaded with calories) than I really wanted. I guess I hoped that somehow it would sink into his tortured psyche that Mom could eat large portions of rich food and stay thin, strong and healthy. But it never registered. How could it? Like anyone in his condition, his brain chemistry had been altered; his brain was being eaten away.

"I'll have the nachos with a strawberry milkshake, please," I told the waitress.

"And, honey, what can I get you?" she asked TJ in a tone that indicated she thought he was 12 years old. In fairness to her, he looked 12 years old. In reality, he was probably older than she was!

TJ: "Do you put grease on your pancake griddle?"

Waitress: "Well, yeah, some . . . so the pancakes don't stick."

TJ: "Oh . . . um. OK, do you have Egg Beaters?"

Waitress: "No, we have eggs, though."

TJ: "Oh, um, no, that's OK. Do you have oatmeal?"

Waitress: "No, but we have cereal."

TJ: "Oh! What kind do you . . ."

I cut him off fuming, wanting to overturn every table in the restaurant! "TJ, enough," I barked. "Miss, he wants to know if you have any fat-free cereal!"

TJ looked mortified. "Mom . . ."

I looked helplessly at the waitress and said, "I'm sorry, ma'am, can we please have a second?" She walked away.

TJ looked so sad, so defeated, so hurt. "Mom, I'm so sorry, I'm ruining your time."

"TJ, I told you to pick the restaurant. I am not going to sit and eat all of this food while you eat a little bowl of cereal and pay a waitress a tip to bring it to us. Cereal is a bedtime snack for a guy your age, not dinner! Let's just grab me a sub on the way home and we'll take it to your apartment and you can have your bowl of cereal there!"

We both got up and put our coats on in silence. I caught the waitress's eye and gave her a silent "I'm sorry" as we left. TJ suggested stopping at a Chinese place instead of going home, and I readily complied. By this time, my stomach was growling!

At the Chinese restaurant, he ordered a steamed rice and vegetable dinner. They quickly served him a large portion—enough to fill two huge dinner plates—and he ate every last bite of it. I was impressed! I would have been pleased had he eaten half. When he was done, I said, "Thank you, honey. Even though it was all steamed and fat free, that was a real dinner."

What happened next shocked me.

We returned to TJ's apartment, bellies full, at about 7:30 p.m. About 15 minutes later, I heard him puttering in the kitchen. I heard the microwave beeping, cupboards opening and closing, silverware clanging, the microwave beeping again. Clearly, he was preparing a meal. How could that be? We had just finished a big dinner! In a few minutes, he came out with a full plate of food, sat down in front of his computer, and focused on his email.

"TJ," I asked, "are you still hungry?"

His silent, almost robotic behavior was my answer. The scene I was witnessing opened my eyes to his particular hell on earth. TJ had become so imprisoned by his own routines that he couldn't break free of them. He had no choice but to adhere to his own rigid schedule—and since he always ate between 8 p.m. and 10 p.m., here he was. At this point, TJ always ate the same things: Jimmy John's fat-free bread, egg whites, carrots, celery, and fat-free cottage cheese, all doused liberally with spices to give the unappetizing conglomeration some flavor. While he ate, he read and answered email, checked his Facebook page, and watched "SportsCenter." But he only allowed himself these rewards if his classes, four hours of exercise, and homework had been successfully completed. On this particular night, in spite of the fact that we'd already eaten a substantial meal and he was undoubtedly full, he was compelled to eat again just to maintain his routine.

I sat behind him on the couch watching him lift his fork to his mouth mechanically, as if in a trance. My heart felt as if it was breaking as I gave in to my fears. I knew for sure what I had been suspecting all day: TJ's obsessions, his rigidity, his inhuman drive had become so ingrained, so severe, that any control he might have had over them was gone.

At about 9:30, he switched gears again and began getting ready for bed. He always turned out the light at exactly 10 p.m. As he hobbled past me, bent over, on his way to the bathroom, he mumbled, "my stomach kills."

For once, I was at a loss for words. All of my common-sense advice, all of my pleas for him to get help, every argument, every word of encouragement, love, and support, all of my motherly wisdom had finally dried up in the face of this unstoppable illness. Nothing came. I felt defeated. I felt the weight of eight years of struggle; of words that were heard but not listened to; of doctors and therapists who tried and failed to help; of trying and doing everything humanly possible to "snap him out of this." I was honestly terrified that the TJ we'd all known and loved, the TJ that the dean had told me to take care of, was gone. I said nothing.

In the darkness, we let silence fill his little studio apartment. I am certain that we both knew what was coming— our eyes were wide open, literally and figuratively. TJ lay in his bed and I lay on the pullout couch. Finally he said, "Mom, I'd give anything to be able to wake up tomorrow morning and have a bowl of cereal with you."

All I could muster was, "Why don't you just do that, TJ?"

"You don't understand, Mom," he said. "Nobody does. Why can't someone just fix this?"

An entire day of held-in tears spilled from my exhausted eyes. I couldn't stop them. They just came and came until my prayers lulled me to sleep.

In the morning, TJ said, "It's gonna be sad, Mom. The next time I wake up in the morning and look over at the couch, you won't be there."

"Awww, thanks honey," I said, still rubbing sleep out of my eyes. "You are the absolute best son I could ever have been blessed with."

13

Merry? Christmas

TJ FINALLY DROPPED the bomb: He didn't want to come home for Christmas. He confessed that he knew he looked horrendous and did not want to spoil everyone else's holiday with worry.

Devastated, I told him that if he didn't come home, he would ruin *my* holiday—that I would have a horrible Christmas if I knew he was all alone in his apartment. And you know what? TJ being TJ, he couldn't bear to make me unhappy. He came home with me.

He engaged in lively conversations with each and every one of his aunts and uncles and cousins, grandmas and grandpas. In addition to our own Christmas get-together, he attended his dad's, his step-dad's and his step-mom's. I don't believe he had ever previously been able to make all four. Some of my family noticed that TJ even stayed up late and played games, whereas in the past he had often escaped to his room to study. All of TJ's loved ones pretended that everything was just fine—but I knew they were concealing their dismay at his appearance, and he undoubtedly knew it, too. Everyone ignored the obvious and we all had a wonderful time. When it was time to take our annual family pictures, I wondered what everyone was thinking, but I also reminded myself silently how lucky TJ was to have such a close and supportive extended family. I have never felt so much love in one room as I did that day.

I decided to embrace the stage we were all in at that moment. Gone were the Christmases with Mom's 18 grandkids tearing open their gifts, flinging wrapping paper everywhere, delightedly shooting Nerf balls out of new toy guns as we grown-ups tried to stay out of the line of fire. Gone were the squeals of my little nieces as they alternately played and plotted ways to convince their moms to let them have a sleepover so the fun would never end. Gone were the days of Grandma Linenger making a delicious multicourse meal for 30 people on Christmas Eve.

This stage was what Christmas should be about—love and family—and I vowed to treasure every second of the day. We were all still together but now the kids' conversations were filled with what classes they were taking at college, what majors they'd selected, what careers they were considering, and who they were dating. I, for one, listened avidly to all of it, fascinated by the hopes and dreams of a new crop of budding adults. How was it possible that almost all of TJ's generation was now college age?

As always, our holiday reunion featured great food; copious conversation; spirited games of euchre, Ping-Pong, and pool; and pretty much nonstop laughter. It was the last time all 29 of us would ever be together, just immediate family and their families—no boyfriends, girlfriends, or fiancés. Just my mom, her five children, and their families. Including TJ. It was a very special Christmas.

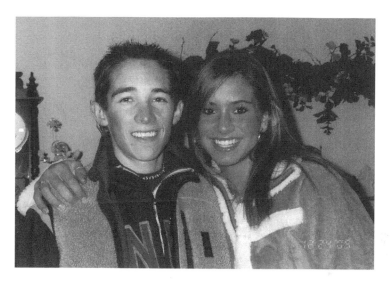

Christmas, 2005

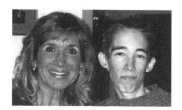

Christmas, 2006
(after one semester away from home with no eyes watching)

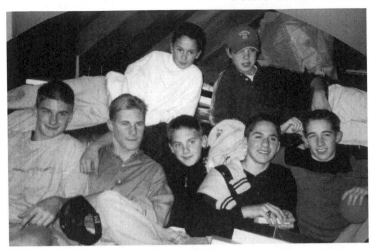

Christmas with his cousins, 2000

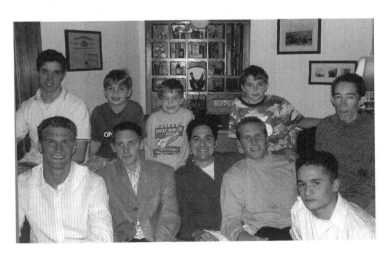

His last Christmas, 2006

When we'd all had our fill of Christmas dinner, TJ volunteered for the job of getting the remaining meat off the turkey. I wish I had taken a picture of the bones that remained. It was funny to everyone else how he managed to tease every morsel off every last bone. To me, it was just another example of his relentlessness. (And of course those bare bones projected an irony of their own.)

What no one else heard was TJ whispering in my ear, "Mom, could you carry the turkey platter to the kitchen for me?" He was too weak to lift it and carry it three feet to the kitchen table. Once the two of us were out of earshot of the rest of the family, I couldn't help saying, "TJ, you just have to go get checked out by the doctor before you go back to dental school. You don't even have the strength and energy to carry a turkey platter! You walk up the stairs to your bedroom like an old man. Something could be very wrong. Please! Let's just go and get you an exam before you go back to school. Please do it . . . for me?"

Amazingly, TJ agreed, on condition we could arrange it for Wednesday afternoon—and it had better not take more than an hour. He had lots to do before heading back to school on Sunday.

I called a doctor friend of ours, Dr. F., who works in the Emergency Room at one of the local hospitals. I told him the situation, and by amazing coincidence he was actually working that Wednesday. I asked if I could bring TJ to the ER because I wanted to make sure that wherever I took him, they would have access to any test or treatment he might need. I knew TJ would only give me one shot.

We walked into the ER and I couldn't believe my eyes! It was packed.

"Wow. No way, Mom," TJ said when he saw the line of sick and injured people ahead of him. "We are outta here!"

"No, TJ, you said you would give me an hour. We're staying for that long, at least. Please sit down."

Sitting wasn't something TJ liked to do, so he stood,

chewing frantically on his gum. (Both burn more calories, remember?) Within 10 minutes, a kind-looking
young intake coordinator called his name in order to get
some insurance information. He also attempted to take
TJ's blood pressure, but had trouble getting a reading.
Looking serious, he tried again—then looked over at me.
I met his gaze but had no wisdom to offer.

"OK, son," he said gently, "let's try rolling up your
sleeves. After trying to get TJ's pressure reading a third
time, he said, "Hmm. That's strange. Wait here, please."

Neither TJ nor I said a thing . . . our minds were too
busy racing. The young man returned quickly and asked
that we follow him past the entire room full of waiting
patients. Several nurses were waiting in a curtained-off
cubicle and one of them instructed TJ to get up on the
examining table. He complained about being extremely
cold.

"Can I have some blankets?" he asked, crossing his
arms over his slim chest. "Or maybe some tea?"

"In a minute, honey," one of them said, as they again
tried to take his vitals. I told him I would be right outside the curtain, a little way down the hall. His panic-
stricken look as I closed the curtain behind me broke
my heart. I was sitting in a chair in the hallway when a
nurse accompanied him over to a scale that happened
to be right next to where I was sitting. He looked at the
nurse and said, "Um, that's my Mom. I don't want her to
see."

"That's OK, TJ. I'll move," I said, getting up.

Once he'd gotten off the scale and set the weights back
to zero, he motioned for me to come back. "Mom, I have
to get out of here! I'm leaving to go back to school! They
cannot keep me here! You can't let them do that, Mom!"

A nurse came over to where we we'd been instructed

to wait and asked me to leave TJ and come with her. She walked me down the hall to where Dr. F. was waiting and as he started talking, I remember the nurse stroking my back. She must have been a mother.

"Susan, TJ's heart is bad. This isn't good. If he were in his 80s, I would tell him he needs to have a pacemaker put in. I'm afraid if he leaves here right now, he might only have two weeks to live."

"Then you must keep him here!" I pleaded, nearly shouting. "You can't let him go, no matter what he says!"

"TJ is an adult, Susan. There's only one way to keep him here against his will and that is by involuntary commitment."

"This isn't going to be easy," the nurse added.

"Believe me, I know," I said wearily. Been there, done that.

"Can you talk to TJ and calm him down?" the doctor asked. "I'm afraid that if he gets all worked up, his heart . . ."

I interrupted. "There is absolutely nothing I can say to him right now that will calm him down. He is going to flip out. He is leaving to go back to dental school on Sunday!"

"Ok . . . do what you can. I'll get the ball rolling."

The next hour was horrible. TJ cried. He accused me of having this all set up beforehand, insisted that I'd tricked him, screamed that he absolutely *would not stay*. He was an adult and legally could make his own decision.

Dr. F. came in and explained the heart results to TJ. "TJ, I want you to know that your mother did not plan any sort of 'intervention' ahead of time," he explained, to my great relief. "As a doctor, I am legally and ethically bound to commit you to a stay in the hospital because I believe you are a danger to yourself and others."

TJ wasn't interested in the test results or the doctor's

concerns. He just sat there stone-faced, repeating, "I have to go back to school. I have to go back to school."

Just a few minutes later, the curtains were thrust open to reveal a uniformed police officer—presumably in case TJ decided to make a getaway. Was I was the only one who could see that TJ was too weak to run? He just looked at me and whispered, "Mom..." We both sobbed.

Reluctantly, I left TJ at the hospital to check on things at home and tell John and Jess what was going on. As I walked into the house and didn't see my husband in his usual spot at the kitchen table, I yelled, "Jess! Where's Dad?"

"I thought he was at the wound clinic," she said.

John had been battling a persistent sore on his hip, the result of friction with his wheel chair, and had been consulting a specialist regularly, including that morning. I looked at my watch. His appointment had been hours ago—he should have been home by now.

Just then, we heard the garage door open and in came John, shouting, "You're not going to believe this! I have to go to the hospital right now because I have an infection in the wound!"

He was right—I couldn't believe my ears. "What hospital?" I asked, numbly, and when he told me I said, "That's where TJ is right now."

This cannot be happening, I thought to myself.

Back at the hospital with John, I felt trapped in a nightmare. My son was on the sixth floor and my husband was on the fourth; both were fighting for their lives.

John ended up in the hospital for 10 months straight. He endured 10 surgeries in 4 different hospitals. TJ on the other hand, was determined to get out of the hospital. He called Dr. F. continually, begging, persuading, wheedling, pleading his case. He got his wish after just two days, having promised the nurses that he would go back to into a residential program. Before going to his room to pick him up, I stopped by the nurse's station.

"I'm TJ's mom," I said. "Your patient with the eating disorder? Are you really discharging him or is he discharging himself?"

"We are discharging him with the understanding that he'll go straight to residential," one of the nurses said.

The look on my face must have communicated my skepticism because she added, "We were in the room making sure he made the call."

"Well, can you officially transfer him there?" I asked. "Just to make sure he goes?"

"Well, actually . . . no," she said, shaking her head. "As you probably know, there aren't any facilities for TJ in Michigan and we're not permitted to transport patients over state lines."

I couldn't even respond. I just turned and walked toward TJ's room, where I found him pacing back and forth, backpack on, ready to escape.

"TJ, what is going on? How is it possible that just two days ago, the doctors were afraid your heart might stop any second—and now they are discharging you? I just don't understand it!"

My mind was racing as fast as my heart. Why were they letting TJ leave? And if he needed to be somewhere else, why couldn't they safely transport him there? After just 48 hours, was he miraculously healed? No longer considered "a danger to himself or others"?

Upon looking into it later, I discovered that they had resigned themselves to simply stabilizing his immediate vital signs. They didn't feel they had any way to treat his eating disorder so there was no point in keeping him.

I picked up his backpack—it weighed more than he did! He had asked the nurses for Baggies and filled them with fresh fruit to take home. "TJ, taking all this food is stealing!" I said.

"No it isn't, Mom; I just took what I couldn't eat so I wouldn't waste it! Besides, do you know how much they will charge us for these two days?"

On the way home, we discussed his plans. He told me that Rogers didn't have a bed available, so he was going to go to school as planned. When a bed opened up, he'd get a ride there.

I was seething. I knew in my heart that this would never happen.

The minute we got home, he went upstairs to pack for school. I reminded him that I couldn't possibly drive him there. I'd just spent a week there, for one thing, and I had his sister Jessie to look after. As if that weren't enough, John was in the hospital, his infection having penetrated deep into his hipbone.

"Don't worry about it, Mom," he said lightly. "I'll call Dad to take me."

About half an hour later, he came down and said in a very quiet, dejected voice, "Mom . . . Dad can't take me. He's going hunting this weekend."

"I am so sorry, TJ, I said," hoping that somehow this would delay his departure. But TJ always managed to achieve his objectives. He went online and made a train reservation. He asked me if I could take him to the train station the next day, Sunday.

That was the second worst day of my life. I watched TJ struggle just walking down the stairs, dragging his backpack. I tried not to look. It was too painful. I felt so

hopeless, so helpless, and so guilty that I couldn't persuade him to get help—or at least drive him all the way
to school. I opened the car trunk and he asked if I could
please put his suitcase and backpack in for him. As he
watched me do it, he said something I will never forget.

"I am so sorry, Mom. This is so embarrassing and stupid that my 55-year-old mom has to lift my luggage for
me. Someday, Mom, I will be taking care of you."

Soon after we arrived at the crowded train station,
we heard an announcement that TJ's train would be 45
minutes late. He immediately insisted that I didn't need
to stay, he knew I had lots to do.

My reaction in that moment felt strange. Half of me
wanted to grab him, hold him, and never let go. The other
half wanted to run as fast as I could, to get as far away from
him and his problem as possible. I could barely look at
him. He looked so bad, so frail. Where did my son go?
The son who could do anything? The son who had goals
and dreams, was full of laughter and fun, valued his health
and strength, treasured his many friends?

We stood there together, making conversation for a few
minutes. He told me that once he graduated, he wanted
me to come out of retirement and be the receptionist at
his dental office. He told me not to worry.

I remember very little from the rest of that day. I think
part of me died when I got to the train station door and
turned to wave to him one last time. I got into my car and
broke down in tears. I don't know how long I sat there
crying. I think I knew it was the last time I would ever see
my son. I almost ran back in, just to get another glimpse
of him—but I knew that the person in that train station
wasn't my son. Some demon had overtaken his mind and
was eating away at his body . . . an outer shell that only
somewhat resembled him.

14

The End

WHEN TJ CALLED me from his apartment that Sunday night, he was very upbeat. He told me that a man in the crowd at the train station had recognized me when I was standing with him, and had approached him after I left. It was an acquaintance from the tennis club. He had introduced himself and asked TJ if he was my son. He was going to Milwaukee, too, and offered to drive him from the train station right to his front door! I was relieved and grateful to have such amazing friends who provided little miracles like this one, helping to keep TJ safe.

On Wednesday, TJ called me at about 5:30 p.m., and this time he sounded upset.

"Hey Mom, wanna hear about my wonderful day?" he said sarcastically.

"Now what?" I braced myself.

"I was sitting in class with all of my friends and all of a sudden two cops and the dean of the dental school appeared at the door wanting to speak to me!"

"What?"

"Yeah . . . unbelievable. They took me to my apartment and said if I didn't open the door they would break it down. They went through my drawers, cupboards, everything."

I was genuinely aghast. "Why? Why did they do that?"

"I don't know, Mom," he said, bitterly. "Maybe they were searching to see if I had any food in my apartment!"

"Then what happened?" I asked.

"The two cops were going to take me back to the residential treatment center. But I insisted on calling Dr. W. on my cell phone. I told him that I needed to stay at school. I reminded him that he knew me well enough to know that forcing me into treatment wasn't going to work."

"What happened?" I asked. And of course I will never understand, forget or forgive what I heard next.

"They left."

I found out later that the police had been called by a concerned doctor at Rogers. TJ made it alone, in his apartment, for six more weeks.

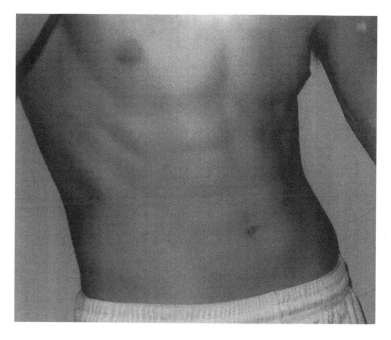

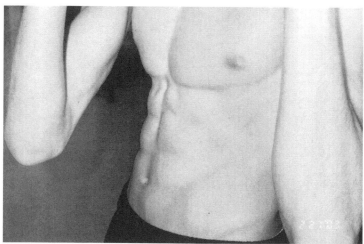

From healthy and disciplined . . .

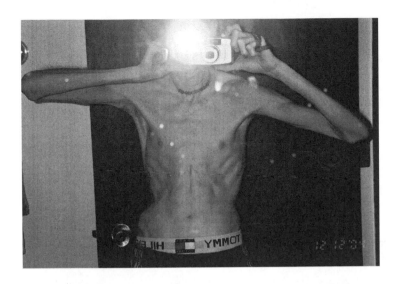

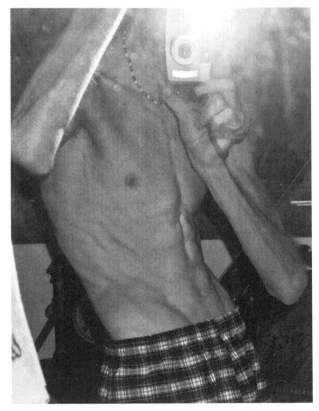

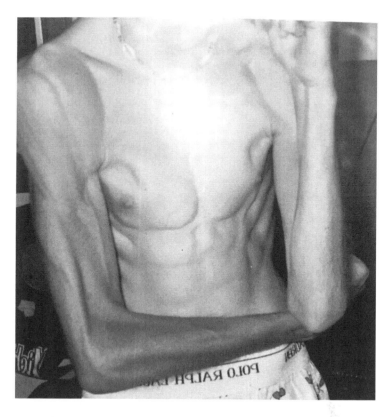

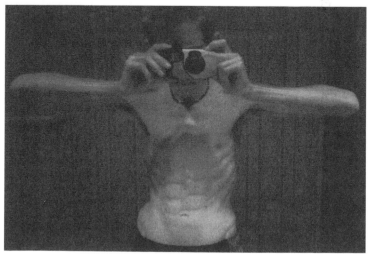

. . . to obsessed and out of control.

The visitation at the funeral home that Friday was a blur. I remember seeing an endless line of people for the entire eight hours, but I can't remember who was there. I remember my siblings trying to get me to sit down or to drink water, neither of which I did. I remember thinking, *Why can't I stop crying? Why am I shaking? Is there a point when tear ducts run out of liquid?* Everyone I spoke to whispered almost the same thing in my ear: "If there's anything I can do . . ."

All I wanted to answer back was, "Yes, there is one thing. Could you please bring my son back?"

Every now and then, I would look around for Jessie, who was hovering toward the back of the room—as far away from the casket as possible. I understood.

To make matters even more surreal, John couldn't be there. He was still recovering from the MRSA infection that had put him in the hospital when TJ was there. In the back of my mind, I wondered whether he would even survive it. And whether I would survive *all* of it.

I knew I had to stay strong and focus on the here and now. I looked at my son in his coffin and thought, *I should have put his newer suit coat on him. This one has a small stain on it. He would not like wearing something that isn't perfectly clean.*

I couldn't help it: I wished I were dead instead of TJ.

Not until you go through a tragedy (or more than one) do you really understand the monumental importance of family and friends. At the end of the night, bone tired as I was, saying good-bye to family and friends in the lobby, my sister motioned me over to join her. We walked back into the room where TJ was and there, in a semicircle around his casket, were 12 of his cousins and his sister. They had all locked arms and were crying. Right there, right then, I realized what life is really about: the unbreakable bonds of family.

Later, I asked Jessie how the 12 of them ended up surrounding TJ and she said, "Mom . . . I don't remember. I think a couple people went up and then one by one we all joined and put our arms around each other . . . I just remember being held up by Bryan."

I will never forget that sight for as long as I live.

When everyone had left the funeral parlor, I went back to say goodnight to my son. I reached down to give him a final hug and broke down. They had stuffed TJ's suit coat with some kind of paper and the crinkling sound almost made me vomit.

The day after TJ's funeral, someone from Marquette called and asked me to come for a memorial service they were planning for TJ. At that moment, I couldn't imagine driving six hours, so I asked them if they could please wait a week or two. They said they'd think about it, and soon called back.

"Mrs. Barry," said a kind young woman from the administrative office at the dental school. "We are so sorry to trouble you, and we can't even imagine what you are going through right now . . . but we feel it is really important to TJ's classmates that we have some sort of service on Monday. They really need to gather together—for closure. A lot of them had planned to attend TJ's funeral but they couldn't get through the snowstorm."

She gave me a few seconds to absorb this and continued, "We'd very much like to make arrangements for you to fly here, if you'd be willing to do that." I was overwhelmed. Of course I agreed to attend.

The memorial service, led by Father Patrick, was beautiful. My heart broke all over again as I watched TJ's fellow students, whom he had so loved and admired, filing into the chapel. It brought back the memory of an ebullient TJ leading me around the school as he told me about each and every one of them.

I burst into tears when TJ's sweet, elderly apartment neighbor hobbled in. She was in her mid-nineties and had taken a bus to be there! She had invited TJ and me to her apartment over Christmas and had told me a little about her life—much of which she had spent in that apartment. When she offered us cookies and milk, I enjoyed mine immediately. TJ "saved his for later."

LAST CELL PHONE MESSAGE

TJ had often asked me not to leave long messages on his cell phone. Instead, he had suggested that I write reminders to myself of what I wanted to tell him and save them for when he had time to chat. I guess that's why I was so amazed by the last message he left on my cell phone. It was the longest one he'd ever left! Part of it concerned his intention to help out his elderly neighbor. He wanted me to be proud of him right up to his last breath.

Hey! I know you're at tennis. I was in the lab practicing for my exam tomorrow morning when you called. I wanted to tell you about my neighbor. Remember that old lady that just turned 95 or whatever? She knocked on my door last night around 7 o'clock. I went to answer it and she was headed back to her room with a bottle of ranch dressing. I said, "Oh, was that you at my door?" She said, "Yes, I had this ranch dressing and for the life of me I just couldn't get it open. Then, as I was waiting for you to come to the door, I somehow opened it. . . . So . . . never mind, but thanks anyway." I said, "Oh, you know anytime for anything like that . . . if you need someone to carry your groceries or anything at all." That was the first time she had come to me. She said, "Oh, thank you so much, dear." So that was that. Then, about three minutes later, there was another knock at my door and it was her again. She had a banana and a can of Coca-Cola in her hand. She just said, "Here, I thought I'd give these to you." I guess she thought I looked too skinny or something. I don't think she would have just come over with a random banana and a coke, but I thought it was a really friendly gesture. So, we talked for a little over five minutes—about the books she was reading, about staying warm, just a really nice conversation. I told her again that if she ever needed anything at all for any reason, not to hesitate to ask me. I thanked her and told her how much I like bananas. So that was my story. I'm probably gonna get cut off but I thought that was pretty cool. I have exams this week so I probably won't be talking to you for a while. Bye, Mom.

At the memorial, there were hugs and tears from his classmates, his professors, and even his former therapist from Rogers. I remember one of the professors whispering in my ear that she was hugging me not as a professor but as one mother to another.

TJ's dad and I went to his apartment to take any valuables before the movers came. I was shocked when we opened the door. His place didn't look anything like it had when I'd been there just a couple of months earlier. It looked like a gym. There were sit-up mats, medicine balls, an exercise bike, jump ropes, pull-up bars, and weights everywhere. Looking at it made me ill.

TJ's father motioned for me to follow him into the bathroom and without saying a word, he pointed to TJ's toothbrush. There was toothpaste on it—all set and ready to go. I just put my face into my hands and cried.

In the kitchen, we found lots of food that he'd hoarded but couldn't eat; we donated it all to a food pantry. One drawer we opened was full of gum, at least a hundred packs.

On his desk was stack of documents. The top one was a letter that the dean had written at his request, in support of his continued attempt to get an Air Force scholarship for dental school.

January 29, 2007
To Whom It May Concern,

I am writing this letter per request of Thomas L. Warschef-sky. I am aware that he is in the Health Professionals Scholarship Program with the United States Air Force. Lieutenant Warschefsky has successfully completed his first semester at Marquette University School of Dentistry and is in good academic standing. He has a perfect attendance record and has completed the first semester of the pre-doctoral curriculum. Additionally, Lieutenant Warschefsky has been elected Treasurer of the first-year dental class and has functioned effectively in this role.

Lieutenant Warschefsky has fulfilled and continues to meet the expectations of a dental student at Marquette. He is a man of integrity and honor; and I endorse him as a continued member of Marquette University School of Dentistry and the United States Air Force.

If you require any additional information regarding Lieutenant Warschefsky, please feel free to contact me. Thank you.

I felt strongly that I needed to talk to the last therapist who had worked with my son. I knew that TJ had really connected with him; he'd told me that the therapist was "a really nice guy, a real sports nut." I was aware that Dr. S. had actually gone to TJ's apartment for their sessions, for which I was extremely grateful. In his weakened state, getting on a bus at dark and traveling to downtown Milwaukee just wouldn't have been safe.

Upon meeting Dr. S., I understood why TJ had liked him. He had a warm face, a gentle voice, and he looked directly into my eyes. As he shook my hand and we both sat down, I could see that he was genuinely shaken.

"TJ was trying so hard to get well, to get this demon out of his head," he told me. "I really feel that he opened up to me and spoke very honestly. He even took me around his kitchen, showing me what he ate."

I'm sure he meant it as a comfort, but what he said next was very hard for me to hear: "I honestly feel that TJ's head and heart were moving in the right direction but it was just too late. His body was shutting down, moving in the opposite direction."

Four years after that meeting, I called Dr. S. again and

asked if he could look back at his records to see if he had any information that might be helpful for this book. He thought for a few minutes and said that he wanted to tell me a bit more about his last few encounters with TJ. He asked if he could retrieve his records, refresh his memory, and call me back, which he did a little while later.

We exchanged greetings and I thanked him for taking the time. "I'm hoping to help other people with this book—I know TJ would've wanted that," I explained.

"I understand completely," he said, with the same warmth in his voice that I remembered from our first encounter.

"TJ had come for a session on January 30, right after returning from Christmas vacation," he began. "Because I knew that he'd been in the hospital, I was especially concerned. TJ told me that he was feeling depressed about his energy level; he just wasn't bouncing back. The following week, on February 7, we had another session and TJ was clearly going downhill. When I brought up the possibility of another residential stay, he wouldn't hear of it. He told me that he'd rather keep working with me on an outpatient basis.

"The next week, he called and said he couldn't see me because he was taking midterms—but he did an interesting thing. He gave me permission to talk with you when you visited him during spring break, which was coming up in two weeks."

I couldn't believe what I was hearing. It was so unlike the TJ who had frustrated me over and over by protecting his privacy so fiercely. "He gave permission for you and I to speak to each other?" I asked. "When was that?"

There was a long pause. Then he said, "I am so sorry, Susan. He called me on February 14th."

That was the day he died.

All of TJ's classmates participated in planting a tree in front of the dental school in his memory. It was a heart-warming gesture, but the other thing they did moved me even more.

Despite their busy schedules, the dental students decided to hold a fund-raiser—a dinner and a talent show—to raise money for the treatment of eating disorders. They sent me a check for $1,000, instructing that it be used to fund an annual race they named 5K4TJ. One of the students designed the T-shirt:

5k4tj
moved by his love, life & spirit

Of course I was delighted to get the ball rolling on a plan I knew TJ would approve of. I expected the first 5K to be very small, but a beautiful, sunny Michigan June day brought hundreds of walkers and runners, and we raised close to $13,000. We combined that with his funeral donations and extended an international grant for $20,000 to

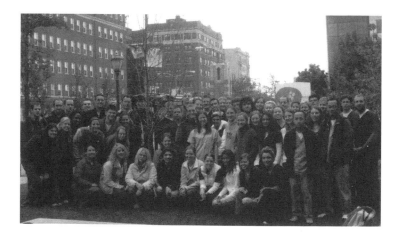

research anorexia with a goal of trying to find some type of helpful medication.

My thinking is this: If scientists can come up with medications for illnesses such as schizophrenia and bipolar disorders, why can't there be something for anorexia? Experts agree that much more research is needed to develop effective and evidence-based guidelines for treatment—but we have to start somewhere, and I was eager to contribute.

In 2010, the mortality rate for eating disorders was higher than that of all other mental disorders put together. Does that give you a sense of how serious this illness is, and how worthy of continuing research?

We live in a society that continues to be obsessed with dieting, weight-loss, and body image. Try channel-surfing or flipping through magazines sometime and notice all the advertisements for exercise equipment, over-the-counter or prescription diet aids, surgeries, and other preparations, devices and plans meant to make us all look like movie stars. The message is all about losing weight—not gaining health.

One of the reasons I decided to tell TJ's story—in spite of the personal pain of reliving it—is that I want to show anorexia for what it is: an illness, not a choice. No matter how strong, motivated, smart, or disciplined an anorexic might be (and many of them are all of those things), this disease cannot be cured by willpower or common sense alone. The love and support of friends and family are important, but they cannot cure it either. More research and more breakthroughs are needed before we can call anorexia a curable illness, but I am encouraged to find that there are more and more professionals every year who are learning to understand and treat it.

As I began my journey through life after TJ, I came

to admire the ingenuity of Elisabeth Kübler-Ross, the woman who came up with the five stages of grief. I also learned a little bit about what one should and should not say to people who have lost their loved ones. I was touched to find out how boundlessly giving, thoughtful and wonderful people can be. But my most meaningful revelation was the understanding of why God allows loss and pain and tragedies to befall us.

So many of us turn to God only when we need Him and get upset when He doesn't answer our prayers. In our despair, we might not even realize that He *has* answered them. There is so much about God's plan that we don't understand . . . especially in times of grief. I have learned now that it is when we are walking that seemingly endless path of deep pain that we learn to feel true passion and empathy for others. The experience of loss instills in us a need to reach out and help others.

One day not long after my son left us, my mom sobbed, "Why didn't God ever answer my prayers? I prayed constantly for TJ. I lit candles, had Novenas said, and asked everyone to pray for him."

I thought about this and only then did I realize how many blessings did occur toward the end of TJ's life:

1. We got to have our last vacation together and his entire family got to share their love with him at Christmas.
2. My sisters were both on spring break and were able to be with me during the horrible week of TJ's death.
3. A blessing in disguise: My mom, who was in her 80s and ordinarily very energetic, had cracked her pelvis while shoveling snow. This meant she was spared the pain of helping to plan her grandson's funeral.
4. TJ made it through Christmas and died where none of his loved ones would have to find him.

5. He chose Valentine's Day to leave us. TJ knew that he could not have been more loved and he wasn't about to let any of us forget him.

6. My dear, lifelong friend was supposed to leave on a weeklong overseas vacation around the time of TJ's death. Her husband got a severe eye infection and they had to cancel their trip, which meant that she could be there with me for TJ's funeral.

7. TJ knew my favorite number was seven. He left me seven emails on Valentine's Day, 2007—the day he died.

8. Another blessing in disguise: Because John was too ill to attend TJ's funeral, we were spared the unpleasantness of his having to be in the same room with TJ's dad.

I think God just couldn't stand watching TJ suffer one more moment, and took him from us as gently as possible. TJ had caused me no pain at his birth and none in the moment of his death. On his tombstone we engraved:

> If love could have saved you,
> you would have lived forever.

I'd like to share with you a little of what I learned about dealing with the grief of losing loved ones. First, it was everyone's sincere impulse to tell me to call if I needed anything. That is more easily said than done. Can you imagine calling someone and saying, "Hi! It's Susan. I was wondering if you could come over and clean my house for me. I just don't have the time or energy." If you want to help someone who is grieving, figure out something they might need and just show up with it. (Think about

TJ's elderly neighbor and her simple, unsolicited gift of a banana and a can of Coke. It is about doing what you can for someone in need.)

I was fortunate to know many people who came over and did things without being called or asked. One day, I came home from visiting my husband in the hospital and my lawn had been cut by a tennis friend. For two months, hot meals arrived for Jessie and me, sometimes stealthily. A big pot of homemade soup would simply appear on our porch with a card, left there by a friend who knew we might not be in the mood for a social call.

I would often find fresh flowers on TJ's grave when I made my daily visit, and found that to be my favorite gesture. In the throes of grief, nothing feels better than knowing someone else is thinking about your loved one, too.

Two very loving friends, Madeline and Julia, started a lunch support group with me. They had both lost children who were in their 20s, too. We met periodically in one another's homes once a month for two years. Of all of my well-meaning supporters, those two were the ones who truly understood my feelings. They had survived what I was going through and were my teachers and mentors. Not a single session went by when I didn't learn something valuable from them. For example, one of them told me, "Be aware, Susan, that when your nephew gets married next weekend, you may not take it well. You could be fine one second, but when you see him standing at the altar, you might suddenly be overcome with thoughts of TJ and all that he is missing out on. You might just break down. You have to remember that this isn't about you and your sadness. It is their happy day and you have to be strong."

I would soon learn just how helpful that little bit of advice would be.

I learned over time that people tend to have one of three very different responses to death and loss, and that these all come out at the grocery store. The first year after TJ died, I tended to do my grocery shopping at 9 or 10 at night to avoid everyone, but inevitably, I crossed paths with friends and acquaintances. Some people would see me and duck into the next aisle. If I caught them at it, I was shocked! Why would they avoid me? Of course I realized later that they just didn't know what to say. They didn't want to say the wrong thing, make me sad, cause me to cry.

Some people I ran into would pipe up, "Hey, Susan! How are you? How's John? How's Jessie? How's Hooper (our dog)?" They avoided the subject of TJ like the plague. Again, they clearly didn't want to upset me.

Finally, there were the people who expressed themselves fully to me. Many of them had experienced loss themselves, so were bolder about broaching the subject. They might say something like, "Hey, Susan. How are you? I think about you and your family all the time. We are praying for you. We have TJ's picture on our refrigerator. We'll never forget that contagious laugh of his. I just can't imagine, Susan. . . ." Then, maybe they would hug me just a little too tightly. We might even cry—but that was okay! It was a blessing for me to hear that somebody else missed TJ, too—and what are a few more tears?

I truly could, should, but probably won't write a second book about death, grieving and the afterlife. Being a Christian, I have always hoped that there is something more than our worldly existence; but to be completely honest, I used to wonder if there really was a Heaven. *Maybe when we die, that really is it,* I thought. Ask me now, however, and I will say that there is no chance that death is the end.

In the year following TJ's passing, I experienced so many signs of his presence that I had to start writing them down. At first, I was skeptical. As a mother, surely I simply was wanting to see signs of him. Perhaps they were all just amazing coincidences. But ultimately, I came to believe that he was really there with me, letting me know that he was happy and at peace.

Loved ones have encouraged me to write about my experiences of TJ's spirit—but I know deep down that skeptics looking for "proof" probably wouldn't believe me anyway. All I can say is that I know, beyond a shadow of a doubt, that I will see TJ again. I am absolutely certain of that.

IF LOVE COULD HAVE SAVED YOU,
YOU WOULD HAVE LIVED FOREVER.

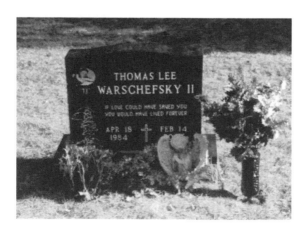

KEN'S LETTER

Often helpful to those grieving is a simple, old-fashioned, handwritten, heartfelt letter. This is an example written by my brother and sent to me two weeks after the funeral when everyone is gone and the house is quiet. Take fifteen minutes out of your day to let them know you are still thinking about them. Reading it made me sob, but it was so worth every single tear.

2/26/07

Hey Susan,

   Out in the world again. People going about their business like nothing has changed. It doesn't seem fair that they can breathe normal, smile without forcing it, sleep more than two hours. They don't understand why I start crying right in the middle of their boring conversation and walk away. It was the same way when dad died. But somehow we go on. I think about Dad every day since he died. I don't picture him with swollen feet when it hurt for him to walk or that forced smile when I knew he was hurting. I picture him throwing knuckle balls that neither Jerry nor I could catch or playing badminton in the backyard while listening to the Tiger game. I picture him playing horseshoes with a beer in one hand while throwing double ringers with the other...bocce ball at Barb's, naps at lunch, driving on vacations—so many great memories. And when I think of them, I take normal breaths. I'm not sure how long that took, but it happened.

   I'm sure it will happen for me again with TJ—not sure if it will for you. You're living everyone's worst nightmare. People will give you all kinds of advice- but no one knows. They all mean well, but your situation is unique. Your relationship was unique. I can't imagine. No one can.

   I'm glad you're there with mom—you guys need each other. I'm glad you were with your sisters. I'm glad I was with my twins and wife. I'm glad Jennie was with Carrie.

I'm glad you have Jess to take care of. I'm glad Tom has Danny. I'm glad TJ has Grandpa.

You've moved to the top of my prayer list. Have no regrets—you were a great mom to TJ. I love you. Thanks for letting TJ be part of my family. Help me TJ. Help me TJ.

Ken

15

For TJ:
A Best Friend's Perspective

DANIEL HOLLANDER AND TJ *met in residential treatment and very quickly became best friends, sharing their
struggles with anorexia and much more. When they met,
Daniel was on his third stay at Rogers; TJ told me at the time
that he was truly afraid Daniel wouldn't make it.*

*Over the years they knew each other, Daniel and TJ opened
their hearts to reveal their deepest secrets, fears, and dreams.
When I asked Daniel what he thought might have caused TJ's
eating disorder, he said he could think of three things: TJ's
relentless drive for perfection; the positive feedback he got
early on for looking "ripped" and "buff"; and his unresolved
feelings about his parents' divorce and its aftermath.*

*Current research suggests that people who get eating disor-
ders are "wired" a certain way. A variety of experiences that
might not be life-altering to others can act as triggers for them.
Perhaps one, two or all three of the factors Daniel mentioned
were TJ's triggers. Perhaps there were others as well.*

*At TJ's funeral, Daniel sobbed over TJ's casket. I put my
arms around him and said, "Daniel, you need to promise me
that you will get well. Maybe TJ died so that you can live."*

Through his sobs, he replied, "I will. I promise you."

*Daniel's road to health wasn't a smooth or easy one. After
TJ died, he returned to Rogers a fourth time and stayed for*

seven-and-a-half months! In addition to his other therapies, he was assigned a private grief counselor. Through his own hard work and the support of many others—and perhaps some luck about the way he was wired—Daniel has so far prevailed over his illness.

Today he is happy and healthy, has a beautiful fiancée, and has graduated from law school. He has kept his promise to me—and I could not be more proud of him.

When Daniel heard that I was writing TJ's story, he asked if he could contribute a chapter. I am extremely grateful to him for his thoughts and unique perspective, and the valuable advice he offers to others suffering with eating disorders. I love Daniel with all my heart—just as TJ did.

I am honored to have an opportunity to tell you about TJ from my perspective, as well as to share my own story of anorexia and recovery. I sincerely hope that it benefits those currently struggling with this devastating and debilitating illness and brings a bit of enlightenment and hope to their family and friends.

It can never be easy to say goodbye to a best friend; someone you looked up too and admired and shared secrets with. It is even harder when you are just 20 years old.

My parents understood how important TJ was to me, so when they received a phone call at 7 a.m. informing them that he had passed away, they got into their car and set out for Washington, D.C., where I was in college, to break it to me in person. Unfortunately, a ferocious blizzard was hammering the northeast that day and they had to turn back home to Pennsylvania. They had no choice but to tell me in a phone call.

Meanwhile, my brother, a medical student in Philadelphia, and my sister, a teacher in New York City, had taken the train to Washington in their place and were waiting at a cousin's house a few blocks from my apartment. Within 45 seconds of my dad uttering the phrase that will echo in my mind for the rest of my life, "TJ has succumbed to his eating disorder," my siblings walked into my apartment to pick me up off the floor and hold me in their arms. Their enveloping warmth helped dispel the hollow pain I felt inside.

A few days later, my parents and I flew to Michigan for TJ's funeral service. I honestly don't remember much of it. I remember feeling numb, shaking, crying, and closing my eyes wishing for my buddy to come back. I am not the most spiritual person, so I couldn't really make sense of what had happened from a religious perspective. All I knew was that my best friend was gone. I felt alone and isolated in a big, scary and unfriendly world.

One thing I do remember from the funeral was the eulogy by Pastor Scott. He explained how awful TJ's death was, and that it might seem as if nothing good could ever come of it; but if someone could learn from TJ's illness, there would be a slight silver lining to the dark clouds surrounding all of us. This was almost exactly what TJ's mother, Susan, had told me the day before at the viewing. As I sat two rows behind Susan at the funeral, listening to the speakers with tears flowing from my red and swollen eyes, I couldn't help but think that both Pastor Scott and TJ were speaking directly to me. More than anyone else in that church, I understood what TJ had been going through in his battle with anorexia. I understood because I suffered from it, too.

It is a strange and terrible feeling to carry the casket of your best friend—especially when you aren't yet even old enough to drink legally. But there I was, on a cold and rainy February afternoon, carrying my best buddy to his final resting place. I couldn't help but think, *why him and not me?* I was confused and angry and didn't get it; how could he have died from this disease? I knew the statistics: One in 10 die from their eating disorder, several others remain chronically ill, and only a few ever fully recover. But these figures had always been abstract to me.

A feeling of invincibility often accompanies an eating disorder (and 20-year-olds tend to feel invincible in any case). Until I lost TJ—someone I knew and loved—I couldn't fully appreciate or believe the statistics. Sadly, I do now.

I first met TJ when we were both patients at Rogers Memorial Hospital in Oconomowoc, Wisconsin. While it might not seem like the most "normal" place to meet a best friend, it shouldn't come as much of a surprise. The people you meet in treatment see you at your lowest point in life. They understand what you are going through better than anyone else can. They are there to pick you up if you start to slip, challenge you, and help you confront the issues that put you there. Ultimately, they are the ones who help you heal and become a better person.

When TJ and I met, we were both on our second visits to Rogers. It was my good luck that I arrived just as a bed opened up in Room 505: TJ's room. We got along right away. It was scary for me to be back in treatment—to admit that I needed help again—but TJ knew just what to say when I expressed this fear on my first night. He instantly put me at ease. The next few nights, TJ and I stayed up into the early morning hours talking about everything. We talked about our particular struggles and what we thought had led to our eating disorders. We talked about recovery. We talked about movies. We talked about basketball and baseball, arguing about whether the Yankees or Tigers had a better ball club (as if there was much of an argument). TJ had a quiet confidence and was a natural leader—attributes that I admired.

It's interesting to look back and realize that within a week of meeting TJ, I knew that I had made a best friend forever, someone who would always be there for me.

TJ was the person that all of the other guys on the unit looked up to. He was funny, athletic, kind, dependable— and very loyal. He made sure that the people he cared about were treated fairly. The week before TJ was to be discharged from Rogers, I was approached by a staff member and told that I would have to move into another room. I wasn't happy about this because it was a hassle, but mostly because I wanted to remain TJ's roommate until he left. I stated my case, pointing out that there was an open room right next door. Before I knew what happened, TJ was upstairs meeting with the manager to make sure that we could continue to be roommates. When I tried to thank him for intervening, he just gave me a look that I knew meant, "Friends help each other out."

Setbacks and relapses are a part of the disease and, coincidentally, TJ and I ended up back in treatment together one more time, both of us in need of a "tune-up." I had been back at Rogers for about two months before TJ showed up. When he walked through the doors, I barely recognized him. He was a skeleton walking. After greeting him, I went back into my room and cried because my friend looked so sick. I was also crying because he probably thought the same of me.

That first night that TJ was readmitted, I sat down with him to discuss his relapse. I was confused because I'd been speaking with him regularly and as recently as a week earlier, I'd been under the impression that he was doing pretty well. I asked him point blank why he hadn't been honest with me. He told me that he was ashamed of his relapse, and he hadn't wanted to admit to himself or anyone else that he needed help again.

"When I found myself lying to my best friend about everything, I realized that I was really in trouble," TJ said.

While it made me sad that TJ was struggling again, a selfish side of me couldn't help but be happy that I had a best friend to pass the time with. This time around, TJ and I were part of a group of guys all very motivated to recover. We tried our best to keep treatment as "uplifting" as possible in spite of the typical drama going on around us. We played games (TJ always won the ESPN board game, except in the baseball category), watched lots of movies, and I introduced everyone to my favorite show, "Curb Your Enthusiasm." Our little group was made up of a unique cast of characters and fortunately everyone got along.

While TJ remained friendly with all of his fellow patients, he approached treatment differently during this stay. Previously, he'd been a cooperative patient, listening to the treatment team and doing his best to avoid bad behaviors, eat what was required, and respect the staff. This time, TJ seemed to have given up.

Looking back on it from a distance of several years, it's clear to me how different his approach really was. TJ was much more combative with the doctors and therapists. He openly refused food and constantly exercised in his room when no one was around. The staff was well aware of TJ's lapses; I saw them confront him more than once, but TJ would simply shrug them off. After staying for only a little over a month, TJ left because he didn't want to postpone dental school. Those of us who cared about TJ expressed our concern that he was not ready to leave. We told him that we thought he had more work to accomplish and school could wait. But TJ could be a little stubborn. He listened to our concerns but said that he couldn't stay any longer. What could I or anyone else have done? It was not up to us.

Before TJ was discharged, we made a contract with each other. We agreed to hold each other accountable and promised to be open and honest about our struggles. We also promised to challenge each other to eat foods that we'd otherwise avoid.

I remained in treatment for another two months but continued to keep in daily contact with TJ by phone, email and text. For the first few months after he left Rogers, it appeared that he was doing well—that our contract was working. TJ was enjoying dental school and was elected treasurer of his class. (This was particularly funny to me since I knew how notoriously frugal he was.)

Unfortunately, as TJ's friends at Rogers feared, his eating disorder symptoms began to worsen midway through the semester. I may have been the one person he was honest with, but even I couldn't convince him to leave school and go back into treatment. He understood the danger of his behavior but still had that feeling of invincibility. TJ made it through the first semester of dental school but by the time he returned for the second one, his heart was irreversibly weakened. He died four weeks later.

People have asked me if I thought that toward the end of his life TJ was intentionally fooling the therapists. Did he *want* to stay ill rather than recover? My honest answer is no. TJ wanted to get better and he knew that he had to if he wanted a future. As he explained to me, no person would trust a dentist who looks like a starving 10-year-old about to keel over.

Yet, even with his desire and motivation to get better, he was unable to do what he knew he needed to do. The eating disorder was stronger than he was and it prevented him from taking the necessary steps.

Carrying the casket of your best friend is even more horrible—and scarier—when you realize that what put him in that casket is the same disorder that you are dealing with day and night. At the time of TJ's funeral, I was relapsing for the fourth time. I couldn't seem to "get it," even with all of the therapist appointments, dietician sessions, and hospital stays. I wanted to be "normal" and rid myself of this awful illness. Before I could, however, I would need to understand the genesis of my struggles.

My struggles with food began well before my eating disorder developed. I was diagnosed in 1997 with Crohn's, a digestive disease. It took doctors quite a long time to arrive at a diagnosis. The one thing I knew was that the pain I was experiencing increased after I ate. Consequently, at the age of 10, I decided that food was the enemy. My mom has told me that she recalls my saying that: "Food is the enemy. I don't need to eat." Clearly, I was terrified of the pain. Even after doctors diagnosed me with Crohn's and put me on a treatment regimen that alleviated the symptoms, the seeds had been planted deep inside me. Food was scary. It was my nemesis.

In the years that followed, I became an extremely careful eater. I avoided certain foods that might be difficult to tolerate and struggled with the fear that at any moment my Crohn's, and the pain, would return. In 2000, during my first year of high school, my Crohn's did return—with a vengeance. I missed a substantial amount of class time because I was always going in and out of the hospital having medical tests. As one can imagine, the emotional toll that Crohn's can take on a young patient is significant. I recall feeling depressed and anxious during the flare-up. My worst fears had been realized: My Crohn's was back. My recovery wasn't easy and took several months, but with the help of new medications, I started to feel better by the spring.

I came to realize that health is a gift and not a right. By late April 2001, I was starting to feel ill again. This time the Crohn's was located in a different part of my digestive tract and in addition to experiencing stomachaches after I ate, it became painful even to swallow food. I went through a battery of tests and again was put on different medications. Additionally, because my body couldn't digest enough nutrients to keep me healthy I was put on supplemental feedings. Each night for six months I had to place a nasogastric tube into my nose and down to my stomach. A machine was hooked up to the tube that provided nutrition all night while I slept. In the morning, I would remove the tube, shower and head off to school. The whole process scared me at first, not just because the tube was horrific in itself, but because food had always caused me pain. The thought of being "fed" all night left me scared and restless, staring at the pump and wondering when the dreaded stomach aches would start. Though my body healed after a few months, the mental scars stayed with me.

The following year, in the middle of high school, another minor flare-up of Crohn's, led me to decide to

take matters into my own hands. I would not rely sole-
ly on medication and good luck to keep me healthy. I
would start regulating my diet. My careful eating habits
morphed into picky ones. I started to question food in
general, wondering how much I really needed. Eventually, it occurred to me that I wasn't just restricting my
eating in an attempt to control my Crohn's symptoms; I
was using diet to control everything in my life. I knew that
cutting back on food would alleviate my stomach pain
but I soon became obsessed with it as a way to control
my life and emotions. The seed that had been planted
in my head years earlier that "food was the enemy" was
beginning to blossom into a full-fledged eating disorder.

Soon, my Crohn's was in remission once more, but
the dieting didn't stop. I was restricting my diet because
it made me feel good—if not physically, always emotionally. Restricting gave me a high and made me feel
accomplished. I felt special being able to restrict my food
intake. I felt in control. At school, I would look around
the lunch table, see everyone else eating, and feel strong
because I did not need to eat.

I discovered that all of my frustrations could easily be
resolved by restricting. If I was angry, not eating made me
feel numb. If I was sad, not eating made me feel better.
If I was anxious, not eating made me feel mellow. Every
emotion I felt offered me a reason to restrict . . . and I did.
By the end of my junior year in high school, there was no
doubt that I was an anorexic.

Throughout the remainder of high school, I was successful in hiding my eating disorder and weight loss. If
my parents or doctors made a comment, I would angrily
respond that what they saw was the result of my Crohn's
disease, and it satisfied them, at least for a while. But at
the end of my senior year, my gastroenterologist pressed

me harder on the subject. I told him that I didn't know why I was so underweight. The truth is, I was genuinely confused. I had never really known much about eating disorders except that anorexia was a "girl's disease." I was aware that my eating habits were abnormal but I never put that label on myself. I never even considered it.

My doctor did—and when he stated his diagnosis, I was outraged. It felt like an accusation. My parents, understandably, were shaken with concern. It was at that moment, just a few short weeks before graduation, that someone had finally called me out on my behaviors— given them a name. Anorexia.

My parents are very proactive in everything, but especially anything related to health. Some might say that they are overprotective—but, as parents dealing with a child who was slipping down the dangerous slope of an eating disorder, they knew that waiting was not an option. Within two weeks of the appointment with my gastroenterologist, they took me to Hershey Medical Center in Pennsylvania to meet with an eating disorder specialist. I hated everything about this. For starters, I wasn't fully convinced that I even had an eating disorder; on top of that, it was my summer break before college and the doctor told me that I might not be able to start school as planned. I fought him hard on this, telling him that a change of scenery is exactly what I needed to get over my "eating issues."

Eventually, the doctor agreed and I was allowed to leave for college in August. In retrospect, I wonder whether I convinced him that this was best for me—or whether he knew that I needed to hit rock bottom before I would be willing to accept help and work toward my own recovery.

If it was the latter, he was right on. My first semester of college was everything it should not have been: lonely,

sad and scary. Continuing my habit of rigorously restricting my diet, my days consisted of only two things:
sleeping and studying. I had no social life because if
I made friends they might want to go out to eat and I
surely couldn't do that. After that first semester, I went
back to see the doctor in Hershey, anticipating an "I told
you so" when he saw me. I was clearly emaciated and my
vital signs were similar to those of an 85-year-old cardiac
patient. In fact, his reaction was more pragmatic; just a
simple but stern message: "The delaying is over, it is time
for you to get intensive treatment now."

As much as I tried fighting, there was no way to win
this battle. The doctor recommended residential treatment and my family concurred. I realized that I didn't
have a choice. I wasn't going to be allowed to go back to
college; my life had been brought to a standstill. After
about a month of trying to delay the inevitable, I finally
caved in and agreed to get help. This decision no doubt
saved my life.

I arrived at Rogers on a freezing and snowy February
morning. I had never before been to Wisconsin, but the
weather was exactly as I had imagined it. Accompanied
by my parents, I checked into the Eating Disorder Center
(EDC) and we met with several of the staff members and
doctors. The whole process was intimidating and scary. I
didn't feel as if I belonged there. The patients I saw were
really sick—that surely wasn't me.

I decided at that very moment that I would do everything I could to get out of there as soon as possible.
With that in mind, I set out to be the perfect patient. I
ate everything on my meal plan from the get go, even

taking optional desserts. I talked about how happy I was to get better and how dedicated I was to making sure I maintained my recovery when I left. I did everything that I thought the treatment team wanted to see. Needless to say, it was all a cover-up. In reality, I didn't want to be there getting help for something that I didn't even acknowledge as a problem. But, I gained the weight and was discharged, claiming I learned all I needed to know. Physically, I was in recovery, but mentally I was still sick. As predicted, it wasn't long before I relapsed and found myself back at Rogers.

It took three more admissions, each ranging from four to seven months, before I finally got to a place where lasting recovery was possible. Rogers started to become a second home to me (not a good thing); I was spending more time there than at my real home! The residential counselors became a second family to me: Mama Cindy, Aunts Renee and Kendra, crazy Uncle Mike. But, while I always trusted them, it was not until my last and longest stay there that I really began to let them into my life fully and let them help me.

Each time I returned to Rogers I learned a lot, believed I was going to be okay, left—and eventually relapsed. I was frustrated and upset with this rollercoaster ride. I felt pathetic. Why couldn't I just get better already?

I recall these feelings coming up a few months after TJ passed away. It was at that point I realized how sick I really was. Having seen my buddy die from this disease, having attended his funeral and carried his casket, if I still couldn't stop restricting, my eating disorder must be stronger than I had ever been willing to admit.

I spoke to TJ's mom and she begged me not to give up and to give treatment another try. She told me that I was the closest thing she had to her own son and she couldn't bear the thought of losing me, too. I heard her words and then thought about my own family. I couldn't bear the thought of them experiencing what Susan was going through. I made the decision to go back to treatment, but this time I was going to beat my illness. I called Dr. W, the medical director at Rogers, and told him I needed to come back.

My last stay at Rogers was also my longest: seven-and-a-half months. This time, I promised myself, I was going to do things differently. I never negotiated my discharge date—I was determined to stay until the day my treatment team came to me and said they thought I was ready to go home. I accepted challenges. I participated in group sessions. I articulated my feelings. I told the staff when I was having urges to restrict and I told them when I did restrict. I was open and honest about everything. I had great support from my therapist, Lee, who worked with me on all of my core issues: fearing how others perceive me, people pleasing, perfectionism, and fear of the unknown (including when would I get sick again). Lee challenged me constantly, which at times drove me crazy and made me want to run away. But this time, instead of keeping my frustration inside as I had done in the past, I shared those feelings with my treatment team. Looking back, I can honestly say that I worked my butt off during that last stay, and that is really a main key to recovering from this insidious illness.

As I write this, my last treatment at Rogers was five years ago. I finally feel like my old self. I laugh. I joke. I smile. I have friends. I no longer fear food and no longer fear Crohn's. I have learned to take the world and its challenges as they come. Most important, I continue to have the love and support of my amazing family and my beautiful and intelligent fiancée, Melissa. I am eternally grateful every day that these people never gave up on me because I recognize now that as hard as this eating disorder was on me, it was just as hard on them.

My journey through the hell that is anorexia was the hardest thing I have ever had to face in my life. My mom always told me that I could beat it and that when I did, it would make all of the other challenges that would undoubtedly come my way that much easier. She was right. But, the truth is, it doesn't have to be as hard as it was for me, or take as long. It doesn't have to end tragically, as it did for TJ. There are ways to help yourself or your loved one beat this illness.

I've thought long and hard about this and have come up with 10 things I believe might help anyone struggling with an eating disorder who finds himself in a residential or inpatient treatment center. I compiled the list based on what I did differently during my last stay, things that helped me finally achieve recovery. Of course, not everything on my list will work for everyone, but I hope it can be a starting point for more thought on the part of all those eager to get well and get on with their lives.

DANIEL'S 10 KEYS TO RECOVERY

1. Don't try to beat the system. My first time in treatment, I did everything I could think of to try to outsmart the team and work around the rules. I knew that in order to be discharged, I had to gain weight and show signs that I was mentally healthy and happy. So I did just that. I ate enough to ensure that my weight gain would be constant and quick. I talked in group about how happy I was that I was getting healthy, how relieved to finally be getting help, and how determined to continue recovery once I was discharged. The truth is I was "BS-ing" my way out. In fact, I was never really comfortable eating what was required nor was I happy to be gaining weight. It was all a lie, a sham, and as a result, I relapsed almost instantly after discharge and found myself back in treatment in just a few short months.

2. Embrace the system. Be completely honest about everything. Don't try to hide what you are feeling or thinking—speak it! The treatment team doesn't expect you to sail through this process without struggles or problems. They know that you might feel angry, scared and anxious at times. It is important that you embrace these feelings and admit to them while in treatment so that you are better prepared to deal with them when you leave.

One particular example of "embracing the system" continues to resonate with me. One night during the first week of my final time at Rogers, they served cheesy enchiladas, a particularly scary meal for me. When I walked in to dinner and saw those large, intimidating tortillas oozing with cheese and sauce, I asked the two residential counselors (RCs) working that evening, Renee and Kendra, if I could speak with them in the hallway. I told them I was not going to eat the meal because I was not ready to take on that challenge. I mentioned that I hoped next month when the same meal was served again, I would be able to conquer it, but that I wasn't quite ready at this point. I didn't know what would happen when I confided in them, and I was definitely surprised by their response. First, they asked me what made it scary and then they asked me to try just a bite of the meal. After telling them again and again that I couldn't, they looked at each other, then thanked me for being so honest. They explained that during my previous stays, I had never been so forthcoming. They knew that I'd confronted similar issues in the past and they were pleased that I was finally ready to be open and honest with my feelings, instead of just doing what I thought would please the staff and get me out sooner. This, they said, was real progress. When we got back to the unit after the meal, the three of us continued our talk about what had happened and marked that meal on the calendar as a goal for the following month.

3. Challenge yourself. While you are in treatment, it is essential to challenge yourself as well as being willing to accept challenges from others. Pushing yourself is really the only way to get better. The challenges you face will be uncomfortable and make you want to quit, but facing them means you are making progress. I was once told by an RC named Mike that treatment should never be too comfortable and that if you are feeling too comfortable, you aren't challenging yourself. He was absolutely correct. So, while you are in treatment, accept every challenge that you possibly can. It can be anything from having an optional dessert each night for an entire week to speaking up more in group. It can be confronting a person in group or going a few weeks without making your bed. Anything that challenges one of your core beliefs or behaviors will help you make progress toward recovery. The great thing about accepting challenges while in treatment is that you are in a supportive environment. If you do become overly anxious or upset while doing a challenge, you have a caring and understanding person to talk with. Challenging yourself while in treatment will help you face challenges after you are discharged.

4. Talk in Group. It is amazing how much you can get out of group if you actually participate. One of the great benefits of group sessions is the opportunity to learn from other people. I bonded over the similarities I recognized between me and my fellow patients—even those who were completely different from me in most ways. They were in middle school and I was in college. They played computer games and I played Frisbee. They watched cartoons and I watched baseball. They cheered for the Red Sox and I cheered for the Yankees. But we had our illness in common, and that meant I had lots to learn from them. The key to a successful group is that all the participants are open and honest with one another. You need to confront each fellow group member in a caring and compassionate way, never attacking or accusing. You also need to challenge one another over problem areas and behaviors. Group sessions become counterproductive when you know somebody is engaging in unhealthy behaviors but don't challenge him. I have been in groups that have failed in this regard, and it only reinforces that person's negative behaviors and communicates to him that it is okay to continue on as before. Even worse, he might come to believe that his fellow group members don't care about him at all.

I understand how difficult it is to initiate a discussion in group. It took me a long time to feel safe and strong enough to confront others. I was always afraid that the person I called out would be angry with me. Eventually, with Mike's encouragement, I learned to speak up. Mike helped me realize that I have a voice and as much of a right to use it as anyone else. He also taught me that if the person I am confronting gets angry or even yells at me, that's okay, too: It's just his eating disorder fighting back. In the long run, speaking in group will make you a stronger person, more assertive, as well as more aware of others' unhealthy behaviors.

5. Talk to the residential counselors. The residential counselors that I had the privilege of working with were the most caring, committed and dedicated group of people I have ever met in my life. More than anything, they wanted all of us to get better and go on to live happy, productive and healthy lives. They were always willing to talk with us and usually had very useful and insightful advice. If you find yourself in a treatment center, remember the importance of having an open and honest relationship with the residential counselors because they will be with you more than anyone else. They are on your side. Seek them out when you are struggling or just need to talk. You will be amazed at how their perspective can make a world of a difference.

6. Use any support available to you. Whether it is your mom, dad, sibling, boyfriend, girlfriend, husband, wife, partner, or best friend, use your support system. It is such a great help to have people you can go to or call when you are having a rough day. Make sure you reach out to someone you know won't be judgmental, someone who is a good listener. You will be surprised how much they can help you. They might offer advice or suggest a different direction. Or, they might simply act as a sounding board, providing you with an opportunity to talk about something totally unrelated to treatment in order to get your mind off of a difficult day or challenge.

7. Trust. It is absolutely, totally, 100 percent essential to have trust while you are in treatment. Trust in the people, the treatment and the need to change. Of course, this is

more easily said than done. If you find yourself in treatment and trust is something you are struggling with, keep
working at it because it is that important. Try to believe
that the people treating you really have your best interest
at heart. They want you to get better. They are not trying
to torture you. How do you establish trust? My therapist,
Lee, helped me with this by telling me that it all came
down to taking a leap of faith. Let me explain. Much of
what your eating disorder tells you is distorted, and while
you may know that intellectually, it is still hard to turn off
that voice in your head and truly believe it. When you
look in the mirror you may see yourself as fat or weak,
and it is hard to believe when people tell you otherwise.
You know what you look like; how can you doubt your
own eyes? This is where the leap of faith comes in. This
is when you have to tell yourself that maybe, just maybe,
you aren't seeing yourself clearly; maybe other people are
seeing you more clearly than you yourself are. Maybe you
really are too thin. Lee taught me to look at it this way:
Either I was right and I was totally fine and everyone in
the world was wrong and conspiring to make me eat and
gain weight when I didn't really need to, or I was sick
and my thinking was distorted and everybody else just
wanted to help me get better. I consider myself a pragmatic person, so when I thought about it, I realized that
everyone else in the world couldn't possibly be joining
forces to make me gain unnecessary weight. This helped
me take the leap of faith and learn to trust that people
did, in fact, want to help me.

8. Understand why you want to get better. A key to getting better is knowing why you *want* to get better. What
is it that you want out of your life? What do you want to
accomplish? Do you want to start a family? Go to college?

Excel at a profession or a sport? Compiling a list of life goals and dreams can be extremely motivating. Equally important is realizing that these goals and dreams can only be achieved by getting better and freeing yourself from your eating disorder.

I worked on my list during my last treatment stay. I still think of new things to add to it. I knew that I wanted to graduate college (accomplished), get into law school (accomplished), and become a lawyer (in progress). I knew that I wanted to make a difference in people's lives, get married, travel the world, have a 7-Eleven Slurpee machine in my house on the beach, and become the starting shortstop for the New York Yankees. I know now that these goals can only be realized if I can stay healthy and out of treatment. (Of course, having the ability to hit a 95-mph fastball would also help with that last item.) Recognizing this was a big turning point for me because I realized I was facing a simple choice: to live the eating disorder life and wind up back in treatment or, worse, dead; or to get onto the road to health and accomplish all of the many goals I have set for myself. When I sat down and thought about it realistically, I was motivated to get better.

9. Be prepared for some turbulence along the way. It is important to understand that there is no such thing as a perfect recovery. You are going to encounter bumps along the way, setbacks, and—who knows?—you might even have to re-enter treatment for a tune-up. The important thing is to avoid getting down on yourself. Don't beat yourself up if you are struggling! Own up to it, be honest with yourself and your support team, and get help right away.

One way to prepare for the turbulence that may come

your way is to make sure you have set up an outpatient treatment team that you get along with and trust. I was lucky to find a wonderful therapist and dietitian in Washington—a husband and wife—Bill and Sandy. They challenged me on my behaviors without ever getting angry at me. They were not afraid to tell me "how it is," and were always able to convince me when the time came that I needed to get back into residential treatment.

Of course it is great if you only have to be in treatment one time before you are able to recover. But if that is not the case, you must remember that asking for help again does not in any way, shape or form mean that you have failed. Recovery is a process that I like to compare to climbing a ladder. You might make it all the way up the ladder without stopping, which is great, or you might have to pause and rest a few times before getting to the top, which is also fine. If you relapse after leaving treatment and must go back to the hospital, you are not starting again from the bottom of the ladder, you are starting from where you left off. So, if, during your first treatment, you make it 80 percent up the ladder of recovery, that means that you only have 20 percent more to learn and conquer before you reach the top.

It took me four stays in residential treatment before I reached the top of the ladder. If I had given up after the second or third time, I have no doubt that I would not be here today. Unfortunately, I know all too well that this does happen. TJ's eating disorder prevented him from going back into treatment when he was struggling during his first semester in dental school. When I encouraged him to seek help, he would say that he had already been to treatment three times and that there was nothing treatment could teach him that he didn't already know. TJ was incorrect in this belief, and tragically, it cost him his life.

10. Give yourself time to relax and be real. Treatment is hard work. Anyone who tells you otherwise hasn't been through it. It is important, therefore, that you give yourself time to relax, laugh—maybe even get into a little trouble. There are lots of ways to do this. You can read, watch a movie, write in a journal, or even play tricks on the staff. It is crucial to relieve stress, at least occasionally.

I used a number of different methods of relaxation while I was in treatment. I watched movies with the other guys and played lots of board games. I also read close to a book per week.

When I was feeling healthy, I even enjoyed "golfing." At Rogers, there is a large, scummy, and deep pond right outside the unit. I would buy 100 cheap used golf balls and, using the club I'd brought with me, I'd tee off into the pond until I was tired. I imagine there are hundreds of my golf balls at the bottom of that pond! When I was feeling a little more mischievous, I played pranks on the staff (many with TJ). While most of them ended with me getting yelled at, they also succeeded in lightening up the atmosphere and making people smile. One of my favorite pranks involved spreading Vaseline on the doctors' doors. Another time, we toilet papered the trees in front of the unit. It is easy to lose your identity when everyone around you is focused on your eating disorder, but remember that you are more than your illness: You are human and you deserve to let loose a little!

I am finishing my third year of law school in Washington, D.C. It has been the most challenging academic process I have ever encountered, and I would not have changed one thing about it. As I spent my nights studying and my weekends locked away in the library, I never complained about the workload. Well . . . not much.

I am thankful for everything I have: the opportunity to learn, live in an exciting city, meet fascinating people, and still have great family, friends and a fiancée to rely on. I realize how close I was to losing all of it. My eating disorder put me on the brink, and I had to fight my way back.

People often ask me whether I would reverse time and change things if I could. My answer is, probably not. Struggling with this illness and spending so much time in a treatment center have taught me more about life than any classroom ever could. I met incredible people during my treatment stays, many of whom remain close friends to this day. I also learned to cherish life because I experienced firsthand how fragile it is. If I could go back in time, it would be for only one purpose: to speak one last time with TJ. I would tell him how important he was to me and how much everyone admired and loved him. He was a leader and wise beyond his years. I will carry TJ's spirit with me for the rest of my life and will do my best to make him proud.

My sincere wish is that nobody would have to go through the hell of this illness. I understand that this is not possible. People will get sick with eating disorders and some of them will die. I do believe, however, that preventive measures can be taken to reduce the number of people who develop this disease. Medical schools need to begin to educate their students to recognize eating disorders earlier. Better treatment methods and earlier intervention would no doubt increase recovery rates. And of course, insurance companies must begin recognizing and covering treatments for eating disorders, rather than proceeding as if they are a "lifestyle choice." They are not.

I did not choose to have an eating disorder any more than I chose to have Crohn's disease.

Eating disorders latch onto their victims and provide them with a false sense of control. Lives are adversely affected at best, and at worst they are destroyed. From my own experience, I believe wholeheartedly that nothing is ultimately accomplished by having an eating disorder. If you are struggling with one, I hope that you discover this fact sooner rather than later so that you, too, can start living the life you were meant to live. Life is too short to let an eating disorder take any of it away. There is too much living to enjoy, loving to share, and happiness to spread.

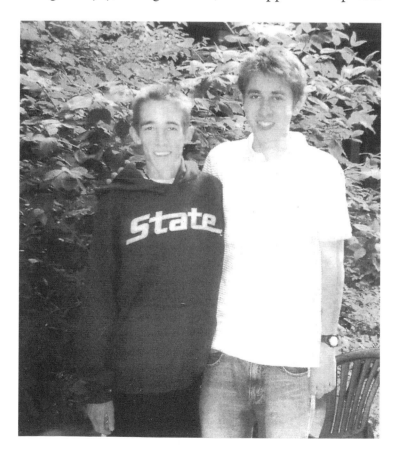

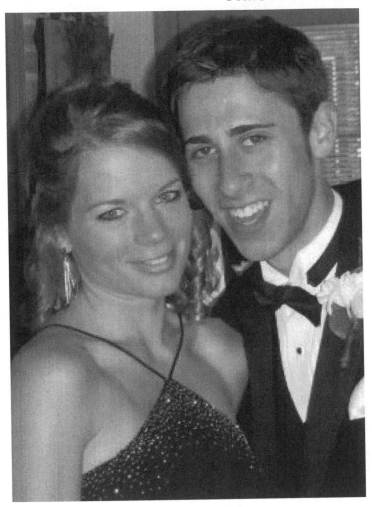

16

Other Perspectives

OVER THE YEARS *he was struggling with his illness, TJ received many letters, cards and emails from family members and friends, all pleading with him to get help. I am sharing some of them here to show how futile words can be—even eloquent, heartfelt ones—when dealing with someone who suffers from anorexia. Some well-meaning family and friends pleaded from a medical standpoint, some from a spiritual one, and still others took an emotional shot at it. We all hoped we could find something new to say, or some new way of saying it, that would maybe, just maybe, reach TJ and help him snap out of his senseless behavior.*

It's important to understand that common sense and pleas—no matter how beautifully stated or how deeply felt—cannot affect the course of the illness once it gets past a certain point. That "point of no return" can't be predicted with any precision, which is why early intervention—going at the problem fast and hard—is imperative.

TJ's father and I divorced when TJ was 4 years old. He wrote this in the process of coming to terms with his son's death.

A FATHER'S VIEW

There are some dates that stay with you. As I write this, it was exactly four years ago today when my life changed. It was morning, and I was ice fishing on a lake in the Upper Peninsula of Michigan while my wife and youngest son were still in the cabin, sleeping. TJ's mom called from her vacation in Alabama and said just two words before she broke down, "TJ died."

What do you say? What do you do? Eight years of battling this disease and watching the changes it made in TJ. Eight years of trying and not trying and arguing and fighting with him and family members about how to deal with the disease.

There's a popular country song called "I Hear Voices." Well, I hear them. Although it is four years since TJ died, they don't go away. When he was alive, I heard the voices of others telling me what to do about TJ—how to change him, how to make him better. They told me where to take him, that I should have him committed against his will, what to give him, what to take away from him. They said that if they were me they would handle the situation differently. Now, TJ is gone and the voices say, "You should have done . . ." and "If it were up to me, I would have done . . ." Will the voices ever go away? Probably not, but they are not quite as loud as they once were.

I have a son!

TJ was our first child so everything was new and special. I thought, *I'd better learn how to deal with baby tantrums because this kid is a handful.* I bought James

Dobson's book, "How to Raise the Strong-Willed Child." People laughed at me and now I chuckle, too.

As I look back on TJ's childhood, I see that he was actually very compliant; he didn't really become "strong-willed" until he was in high school and college. I was proud of my son, of his personality, his scholastic and athletic achievements, and the fact that he was such a nice kid. Everyone liked TJ. He was polite, honest, industrious, friendly, and able to relate well to everyone from adults to toddlers.

So much of that changed as his disease progressed. On the "outside," he still had all of the positive attributes— but to those closest to him, he changed. He became secretive, moody, and lied to cover up his exercise activity and eating habits. He became controlling and manipulative. TJ wanted to be in control of his food, schedule, activities, and finances, even if someone else was paying for them. He had to have a single room on campus so that he could study and he continually promised that he'd gain weight if only I would keep paying his college expenses. He negotiated with me over buying his foods of choice, telling me that they were the only things that could help him gain weight. Instead, he'd lose more.

The arguments over what to eat and how much to eat seemed endless. Through four years of college, he bargained with me to support him financially and physically and help him stay on his scholastic schedule. We argued about whether he would exercise and how much, and about which family functions to attend. My background in nutrition only made his behavior harder to understand because the numbers are simple. To gain weight you must put in more than you use up! At times, he would reluctantly accept help and counseling or rise to a challenge, deadline, or threat to withhold finances or privileges. But for the most part, he did exactly what he wanted.

What do I think about? The total frustration and helplessness I felt when nothing seemed to work. I think about how I could never understand how something so intangible could have so much control over a young man's life. How could the solution to his physical problem be so simple and yet so difficult to make happen?

"What's wrong with you? Why don't you try? Can't you see what it's doing to you and your family and all of your relationships?"

It just didn't make sense to me that someone who had always been so eager to please had become so difficult to reason with. Was it just because he was growing up and making his own way? Was he just becoming his own person? It's not as if he was smoking or doing drugs or getting drunk or sleeping around. Lots of kids do those things in the course of their college years. This was different—or was it? TJ's actions must have been affected by typical peer pressures as well as the burden of having divorced parents and stepfamilies.

Did TJ's illness develop because we got divorced when he was 4? Was it because each of his new families went on to have another baby and he was no longer the only child of either of us? Did we expect too much from him? Did he feel extraordinary pressure to excel?

It's easy to assign blame to one factor or another. Perhaps his personality made him particularly susceptible to this condition; maybe his problem was exacerbated by ignorant or inept counselors, doctors or administrators. Maybe his family and friends failed him by trying the wrong things—or not trying hard enough. But in the end, what good does assigning blame do for TJ or the loved ones he left behind?

During his last Christmas break in 2006, TJ pleaded and guilt-tripped me to try to get me to take him back to dental school. At that point, our relationship was strained. I had asked him earlier in December if he would go for help over Christmas and he had said there wasn't enough time. While he was home, he didn't go to all of my family gatherings. After some argumentative phone calls, he finally admitted in an email that it was hard for him to get together with people because of their reactions to how he looked. One of his journal entries from that time reads, "I have dug my own grave though, and I'm about 5 feet under. I am so ashamed, mad, disgusted, embarrassed, you name it. . . . I want to curl up in a room and just feel sorry for myself, but I need to face reality and deal with it b/c it's my own fault, and I have to get myself out of what I started."

There were only certain days I was able to take TJ back to school, and I was not feeling very charitable. He insisted on a particular day and I said no. He left mad and took a train.

We exchanged a few cryptic emails over the next six weeks, mostly about the weather, his classes, and what was going on with my business.

Was there a point when he lost control of his actions altogether? In my view, it wasn't a point in time. Rather, the disease gradually took over. You could say he was making choices about what to eat and how many sit-ups to do each day—but really, he just wasn't in control. He was aware of the pain and discord he caused within his family and yet he chose to continue his downward spiral—or did he choose?

TJ rejected counseling and medications. He agreed

to inpatient treatments at various points, but only under his conditions. He even convinced the professionals that he should be allowed to do things his way! He thought he was in control of his life, *but the disease was in control of him.*

What would you have done if you were me? Maybe your situation is similar, and if so, you should know that you are not alone. Thousands of people are diagnosed with eating disorders every year, and many more go undiagnosed. Too many of them die, though many do not. Why did we lose TJ? I ask myself that every day.

At this time, there are many more questions than answers about anorexia, but important research is in progress. If you'd like to support this work, please check out TJ's Fund for Eating Disorder Research *and feel free to make a donation.* Just go to www.aedweb.org and click on "Get Involved," "Donate," and "TJ's Fund."

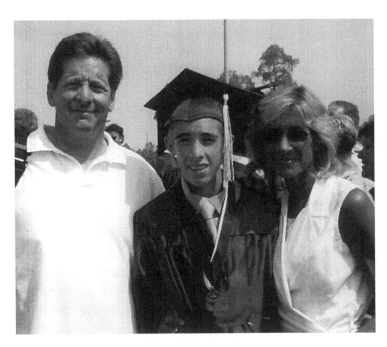

A STEPFATHER'S VIEW

TJ came to be my stepson when he was 5 years old, and right from the start, we had a great relationship. He was a fun and happy kid. We played chess, checkers, euchre, and lots of board games together. We wrestled on the floor and I "tickle-tortured" him. Like me, TJ loved to eat and ate everything and anything.

As he got a little older, we spent hours working on his sports skills. He could really dribble that basketball, even spin it on his fingertips, and once sunk 32 free-throw shots in a row. We'd toss the football, play floor hockey, and play catch with a baseball. He took on my absolute love of Michigan State basketball and was always looking for the latest news flashes about the Spartans to share with me. Because he had a steel-trap memory, he excelled in sports trivia and we had fun quizzing each other.

As TJ entered high school and his eating disorder began to take hold, our relationship became strained. I was a teacher of the emotionally impaired, and changing bad behaviors was my area of expertise. It became very frustrating to me that none of my tried-and-true techniques seemed to work . . . or not for very long.

TJ's illness changed our family dynamics. He wanted his mother all to himself, to talk only to her and do things only with her. Susan constantly found herself torn. If we went out to a restaurant, Susan was afraid that if she sat next to me or Jessie, TJ would get jealous. In family pictures, TJ had to stand next to Susan. Too often, it felt as if TJ was manipulating and controlling all of us. And his dependency on Susan didn't seem natural.

TJ's inability to spend any of his money was frustrating, too. It wasn't until late in the game that I realized this was a symptom of his illness—another area in which he exerted obsessive control. His strict routines and schedules seemed to get more extreme over time. As the anorexia gripped TJ more tightly, the stress level at home increased. It was so difficult for all of us to watch a once fun-loving, happy, social, and content TJ turn into someone we didn't even recognize.

It didn't happen overnight, but he seemed to keep setting the bar higher (meaning lower) each time he accomplished a goal. If he weighed 105 pounds, he decided to try to get to 100. When he did that, the goal became 95. Then he vowed never to go back to weighing a three-digit number. He cut out fat. When he'd accomplished that, he took sugar off his list. Eventually, he'd eat no food with calories. He'd do 500 sit-ups per day. When he'd mastered the task, he upped it to 1,000—and then 1,000 in the morning and 1,000 at night! He never let up on this routine, even when he developed a painful cyst on his lower spine. Exerting this kind of control over himself made him feel powerful—but sadly, whatever he accomplished, it was never good enough. Stopping was not an option. Doing less was not an option.

What would I have changed, knowing then what I know now? I would have tried to understand better what TJ was going through and stay closer to him. I would have worked harder to keep our lines of communication open. Throughout his illness, I was dealing with my own—multiple sclerosis—and I thought that being a good role model would help TJ. I never, ever believed he would die from this.

I applaud my wife for writing this story, as hard as that was to do, because I know it will help others. I think that by getting to know TJ, people will understand that anorexic behavior isn't a choice and it isn't something that one can just stop. TJ's drive and perseverance were unmatched, but he could not get off the self-destructive path he was on.

I have been told by many people that my patience is unmatched, but dealing with TJ's illness put it to the test. I empathize with any parent having to deal with this insidious disease and hope that you can somehow find the strength and patience you will need.

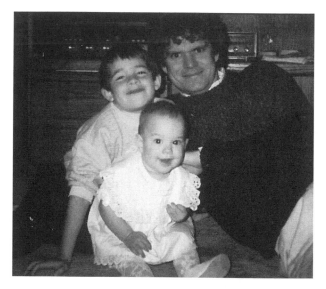

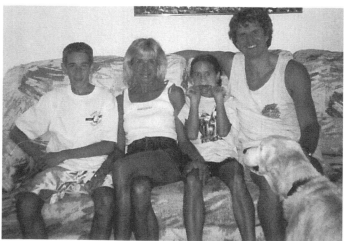

A GIRLFRIEND'S VIEW

Ashley Scott was TJ's high school girlfriend. I will forever be grateful to her because she is probably the only girl that my son felt that heart-fluttering love for. I am so glad he had a chance to feel that. Here's Ashley's perspective, beginning with an excerpt from an email she sent to me.

This was s o hard for me . . . I don't know how you wrote all of those other chapters. I can see how this would totally consume you. Even after all of the things I wrote, there are still a million thoughts swirling in my mind. When I read what I already had written, I kept thinking, "That isn't expressing the devastation I felt when I saw him looking so sick, or the disappointment I felt when he put everything else before me, or the j o y I felt that one Christmas when I came over and he looked so healthy".

Lots to tell you.
Lots of love to give.
Lots of laughs to have.
Lots of time to make up.
I do love your guts.
I tried not to love you, but it is not up to me.
There is something bigger than me that makes me love
    you.
Serendipity
Teej

Those were the last words TJ wrote to me after having the fight of all fights. It was the letter I had been wait-ing for throughout the previous few months, after the summer of hell. It makes more sense for me to start at the end rather than the beginning, because it wasn't until the end that everything started making sense and I started putting the pieces together. All of the mistakes I made, all of the opportunities I let pass by, all of the things I didn't say, and all of the struggling I didn't understand... none of it was revealed until it was too late.

Senior year was when I started realizing who I was and the kind of person I wanted to be. I figured out who my friends were and the types of people I wanted to surround myself with. One of those people was TJ. In my eyes, TJ was perfect.

Throughout our senior year, TJ and I spent a lot of time together and created countless memories. I never thought I would be looking back at those memories trying frantically to remember every single second. The first time we went out together was to an MSU tailgate. I was starving, and looking forward to a hotdog, chips, cookies, and everything else that goes with a football game. Hot dog in hand, I asked TJ what he wanted, and he said he had eaten earlier that day and that he would just snack on the vegetables. Constantly being around a lot of girls who skip lunch and talk about how fat they are, I was instantly embarrassed that I was eating a hot dog. That was the last time I ate something unhealthy in front of TJ. I wanted him to think I was as healthy as he was ... or as healthy as I thought he was.

We used to walk around the campus of MSU eating Baskin-Robbins. We would order the same thing: nonfat yogurt with strawberries in it. We would eat sandwiches at Jimmy John's—day-old bread and veggie sandwiches with no dressing. We would go out to dinner and TJ would order a salad with fat-free dressing. The entire time this was happening, I was completely oblivious to every single effort TJ made to avoid fat. Rather than noticing it, I conformed to his eating habits. Like I said, I wanted him to think I was healthy and in shape. Of course, TJ and I couldn't do any of the activities mentioned above until he had worked out for hours. I waited.

As we spent more time together, I started becoming more self-conscious because I didn't have the discipline and control that TJ did when it came to exercise and eating. On top of that, TJ was hesitant to invite me over to his house, so my feelings got hurt. Why didn't he want me to spend any time with his family? In my confusion, I began to pull away. My mind went everywhere else except what now seems like the obvious place. TJ did not want me to become close to his family because he was afraid I would discover his secret.

The school year came to an end. While I was enjoying my friends and family at my graduation party, I kept wondering why TJ wasn't showing up. Later, I learned that he was being forced into a van against his will and taken to a hospital. We had just had our picture taken together a couple of hours prior to that.

I never imagined TJ to be anorexic. I was envious of him and wished for his skinny legs and rock hard abs. Even during freshman year of college, when rumors started to fly that TJ was in residential treatment, I didn't get it. I called and emailed him to see if he wanted to meet me in Okemos one weekend. He said he had a cross-country meet and I didn't know what to believe. I never thought TJ would lie to me, so I ignored the rumors until they became difficult to ignore.

When TJ had canceled plans a few too many times, I began searching deeper and finally connected with his mom for clarification. She kept TJ's secret for the first couple of months, and then eventually the truth spilled.

TJ would have been devastated to know that I knew everything he had been hiding from me for so long.

TJ and I continued to spend time together throughout college. I would go to Albion and he came to Holland. The weekend he came to Holland, I bought all fat-free food for my dorm room: vegetables, fruit, rice cakes, and gummy bears. At that point, TJ wasn't counting calories yet, so anything fat free was fair game. Though I was enabling TJ's habit, I truly felt I was being a good friend. I kept his secret, even from him.

When I think about TJ now, I think about the memories I have of him when he was still himself. I don't feel comfortable saying he was healthy—but he was trying. There are two vivid memories I will never forget. The first was when I went to pick him up from Albion to go back to Okemos. We both wanted to go home for the weekend, so I drove from Holland to Albion. When TJ came out to my car, I wanted to start sobbing. His skin was pale and sunken in, his hair was thinning, and he looked worse than I had ever seen him . . . worse than I had ever seen anyone. It was the perfect opportunity for me to initiate a conversation about his illness. I ignored the obvious, once again, held his bony hand, and drove in silence most of the way home. It wasn't too long afterward that he was back in treatment.

Finally, the time came when TJ knew that I knew about the eating disorder. I don't remember the specifics of how that was revealed, but it was Christmas and we went to the Potter Park Zoo for the holiday lighting display. He had just come home from being in treatment and he looked like himself again. He had regained his sense of humor, he looked healthy, and everything was right in the world again. I will never forget my feeling of relief when I walked through the door and saw him looking so happy. As we walked through the park, I remember squeezing his hand and simply saying, "I just want you to be OK. I'm always here if you want to talk but I'll never ask you to." All I wanted was his friendship and for everything to go back to the way it used to be. For a while, that was exactly what happened, until he started falling back into the same routines.

Eventually he became wary of my spending time with his family. None of us knew how to help TJ, and in the midst of the battle that everyone wanted so desperately to understand, he began to push away from the people who loved and cared about him the most. Eventually, TJ made me choose between my friendship with him and my friendship with his family. I chose TJ, but I became angry and resentful. I did not understand how someone could be so stubborn and selfish. We began lying to each other and I spent time with his mom behind his back. He stopped talking to me completely.

That summer, I wrote him an email every single day. I didn't care if he answered them—but I wrote them. I left things for him at his house, notes and gifts. Eventually he responded with an email to apologize to me, but also to explain that he did not want me communicating with his family. In the middle of a single-spaced, four-page email, he wrote. "I want to tell you *everything*. I want to pour my heart out to you, but I don't feel like I can tell you what I did yesterday without you telling my family." If I were going to be on his side, as I had claimed to be, I had to discontinue my communication with them, and not talk about him with them at all. I basically needed to stop trying to help.

That brings me back to the beginning of my story: the last words he wrote.

I will never be able to share all of the stories, experiences and emotions that made up my complex relationship with TJ. If anyone were going to be able to overcome this, it would be TJ . . . all he had to do was set his mind to something, and he could achieve anything. People always say grand things about those who have died, and sometimes they embellish the person's qualities. TJ truly was one of the most honest, genuine, loving, incredible people in my life, and I consider myself very lucky to have had him as my friend.

We never got to do all of the things we talked about doing together or fulfill all of the plans and adventures we conjured up. TJ's life served a purpose, though, and so did his death. Although I do not understand how such an incredible person was robbed of a long and healthy life, I try to find comfort by believing that he was meant to do something bigger.

I don't know if I will ever truly understand . . . but there is not a single day that goes by that I don't think about him, and wonder what in the world I could have done differently.

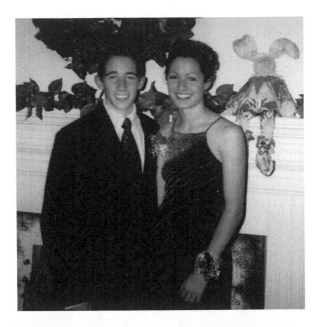

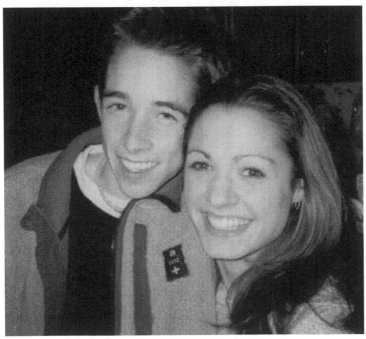

A COUSIN'S PERSPECTIVE

Here's an email exchange between TJ and his cousin after they saw each other at TJ's last Christmas with us, in December 2006.

TJ:
Hey Man,

Good to see you at the Linenger's, is everything all right?

You seemed to be a little down when talking to me . . .

Rhett:
Well, I didn't mean to be down, but if I did seem to be it might be because I know how much potential you have and how smart you are and it really bothers me that you are still doing this to yourself. I know what you are capable of and so do you, but I don't think you will be able to accomplish the things you are capable of accomplishing if you keep this up. I don't want to be going to your funeral in the next 10 years, TJ. I don't think I have ever been this blunt about it because I didn't want to offend you, but there is no point in me not telling you exactly what I think. I KNOW you are mentally strong enough to beat it if you want to and it bothers me that you haven't. . . .

Well, I didn't mean to come off down and I wasn't going to say anything but I guess if you could tell that something was bothering me, even with me trying to cover it up, it is worth telling you what was bothering me. TJ, I see us as being very similar in almost every way, intellectually, the way we love sports, our work ethic, our drive to succeed, and I don't see that in a lot of other people. So it really bothers me to see someone close to me doing things that won't let them reach their potential. Maybe you will be able to get there and keep this lifestyle, and I H O P E that is the case. I just don't T H I N K it will happen that way and I'm sorry, but that is the way I feel.

TJ:
Hey.

Thanks for being honest. I'm not mad at you at all for being honest with me. I would rather you tell me like you did in the email, than just have you going around feeling like you did and not able to really talk to me about anything. I know it's got to be frustrating for you to see me like this because you know how I looked when I had about 40 lbs. more of muscle on me and everything. You have no idea how embarrassed I was to come home for Christmas and see all the family. My mom basically had to beg me to go. I know that I can never be a dentist looking like I do—who would trust somebody to take care of them when they can't even take care of themselves? I know I can't do this for three-and-a-half more years in school, too. To be honest, you are really a good motivator for me when I see you. Not to be gay or anything, but you're obviously built like a brick house and you have good looks—both of which I know that I could have, too, if I just ate more and exercised less. Seeing you gets me pissed off at myself and motivated to eat more and look good again. Hearing you talk about lifting/eating/playing sports does the same.

It really isn't about W H A T I eat anymore—the problem is that I don't eat enough calories and I exercise too much. I have gained weight and been at a healthy weight eating my fat-free stuff. I just have such a hard time with a long-term motivation with this thing—which is completely opposite from everything else in my life. I feel motivated for a day, week, couple weeks, and can put weight on . . . but it invariably seems to fizz out and I revert back to the bad habits. It is so weird to me that I can accomplish almost anything I set out to do but this hangs me up so much. I guess it's because the weight/not eating thing is in my head as a sign of discipline and determination. So keeping the weight down, or not eating, or exercising, shows/proves to myself that I am strong (yes, I know you are probably thinking: "so just turn it around and say that gaining weight and eating are what really would show the determination." But it is not that simple!)

Anyway, I know you are busy so I won't drag this on. Thanks for telling me how you really feel about it. I wish there was a pill I could take that would put 45 lbs of muscle on me overnight, but I gotta do this for myself—and do it quick.

Good luck this semester. I can't believe the Lions won today—they just blew the #1 pick!
TJ

I received this email from a college student I was trying to help. I am including it because I believe her words express a very common feeling among anorexics and reveal a little bit about how their minds work.

Dear Mrs. Barry,

I so badly want to say something to my Dad right now and don't want to wait another minute. But I just got out of inpatient care and going back to treatment would mean that I am admitting defeat. I am just scared and don't know what is the right thing to do. ED (Eating Disorder) is making me feel like I am doing something right because I am losing weight again. Even though I still feel fat, I can see my bones even more and it just gives me a sense of success. It is like a false sense of happiness.

Not having a scale and weighing myself 24/7 makes me feel like I could be gaining weight. So, since I don't know, I assume I am gaining weight and I lose weight. I would rather die than gain any weight. That is how unhappy I am with myself and if my control is taken from me again (or from ED, rather) then it makes me feel out of control and not having something to control makes me so unhappy.

I lost my mom and grandmother and it feels like my world is spinning out of control and food is the only thing I have control over. Yet, at the same time, it is like I really don't have control, because ED really has the control and I am scared to make "him" mad again. I just don't know what to do. I hate being dishonest with everyone. It is NOT who I am! I just can't help it.

I don't know if I would hurt everyone even more by going away to residential. Like, will everyone think I am a failure or that I just like the attention when I really don't want people to think that? I know deep down it is what I need, but ED really doesn't want me to admit it. I am afraid to admit it because I feel everyone will think it is some cop-out to get out of real life when the life I live now really isn't a life. It is a disease that is destroying me.

I am just so lost and confused and hanging on to my eating disorder is all that gives me purpose in life. It is who I am and without it, where does that leave me?!? I am numb inside to true feelings. I don't know what it is like to live a life without an ED. I have lived my whole life like this. It isn't right for me to be afraid of food and being at a normal, healthy weight, but I don't know what to do about it. I guess because I feel so fat and disgusting that until I get back to that brink of death, I will never feel satisfied with myself or my body—even though, THEN I wasn't satisfied either! I felt HUGE at 85 pounds. I would have died if I hadn't gone to treatment. Sometimes, it almost feels like it would have been worth it because of everything I have been through.

This road to recovery seems a lot harder than I thought. Fighting makes me scared, but not fighting makes me scared, too. I don't know what I want or what is right anymore. At first, I could distinguish ED's thoughts from mine. Now I don't know what is real and what is fake.

17

TJ Speaks

AT THE END of the three months of residential treatment, TJ had gained almost 30 pounds. It was amazing to see his personality, sense of humor, and joy return—he was the old TJ again! His skin had a healthy color and the sparkle returned to his blue eyes. He started laughing again and so did I.

While in treatment, TJ wrote several poems, kept a journal and started writing a book. At a more normal weight, he appeared to become a rational thinker again.

In this poem, TJ's restored sense of humor is evident.

FAT

Fat is butter, fat is meat.
Fat is something you must eat.
Without fat you're always cold
And often feel weak and old.
Everybody needs some fat,
Without it you are thin and flat.
If you don't eat fat and lard,
You're pooped and cannot mow the yard.
Without fat you are always tired,
Your performance sucks, you might get fired.
You don't want to have fun and play,
You just obsess on food all day.
You get depressed and have no fun,
You never go out in the sun.

You cannot run, nothing gets done,
You have no buns, and that's no pun!
You never sweat, you never smell,
Your life is like a living hell.
Your heart slows down, it may just stop,
And all you want is diet pop.
When there's no fat, you cannot dump,
And in the mirror, you have no rump.
Standing up can make you dizzy,
You always have to feel so busy.
You have no fat, it hurts to sit,
You feel sad, your clothes don't fit.
Without some fat, you'll lose your hair,
And having fun gets really rare.
You lose your family, lose your friends,
The lies you tell will see no ends.
Without fat it is hard to choose,
You never win, but hate to lose.
So eat some fat and gain some weight,
Before you die and it's too late.

This is a reflective poem about wanting his old self and life back.

Remember When . . .
(05/16/05)

Remember when you used to laugh and always be so
   happy, and when you didn't feel like your life was so
   dang crappy.
Remember when you used to have a hundred thousand
   friends, the fun you had in high school just seemed to
   have no end.

Remember when you used to hunt and fish and ski out
west with dad, or when a change in schedule wouldn't
make you get so mad.

Remember when you used to be the best at every sport
you try, or when you used to be so moral, and never tell
a lie.

Remember when you used to have the girls always calling,
but now you've tripped and lately it seems like you
can't stop falling.

Remember when you used to be the model "perfect son,"
you worked so hard, but always made the time to have
some fun.

Remember when you used to be so strong and very buff,
for all you had you never were content with just that
much.

Remember when you used to have the greatest sense of
humor, but now you look as though you're dying from
a tumor.

Remember when you used to reach your every single goal,
your eating now has put you in a deep and dirty hole.

Remember when you used to NEVER argue with your
mom, but now you guys yell and scream, exploding like
a bomb.

Remember when you decided that you need to change
your ways, you realized that being healthy will bring
many happy days.

His fears are still apparent.

Untitled (5/19/06)

If someone wrote a script of where I'll be a year from
   today,
I wonder what my plans will be and just what they would
   say.
I have my hopes, I have my goals, and surely have my plan.
But will those dreams be realized or will they hit the fan?
I want to go to dental school and right now I'm applying
but next year will I be accepted or will I be found crying?
I wish I had decided on my future much more early,
cause now I'm playing catch up and that I know will hurt
   me, surely.
Today I'm at the EDC and trying to gain some weight,
will it last, will I maintain, and will I have a date?
I wonder what will happen when some things don't go my
   way.
Will I relapse, will I stay strong, and what will others say?
If I could make my perfect plan of just where I would be,
I don't think it will happen, but I'll write it just to see.
U of M, Nova Southeastern, Colorado or UNC,
Each of those would make me just as happy as could be.
If I don't get into dental school I wonder just what I'll do,
I do not want to live at home, but that I already knew.
Will I take a year off and study and reapply
or will I give up and not even give it one more try?
Will I change and go into law or get an MBA,
will I get an internship or short-term job for pay?
I haven't been in contact with friends from my senior
   high,
I isolated and now it seems like those years just flew by.

I hope that we can get back together and maybe just hang
out,
I'm embarrassed to call them even though they'll take me
back . . . no doubt.

And of course, this one is my personal favorite.

Mom . . .

18 years have come and gone as quickly as I came;
Many things have happened since but you remain the
same.
We've laughed & cried, we've played & worked,
we've gone through a divorce;
But over the years my love for you has grown with so
much force.
You've always been there to give advice and
help me when I'm down;
That smile of yours is strong enough to wipe off my lon-
gest frown.
An "Athlete," a "Teacher," an "Advisor," a "Friend";
The perfect "Mom" whose wisdom and love has no appar-
ent end.
I know that you're perfect, I mean, sure, you talk too loud;
But when asked if I am "Susan's son," I feel so very proud.
And maybe you sometimes give one or two [too] many
suggestions;
But in the end I realize, they're all good life-long lessons.
Getting ice cream at Baskin-Robbins, playing tennis, or
taking a run;
These are some of my favorites with you,
but you make everything else so fun.
I'll never forget our spring break in Florida and driving

across the whole state;
Or the look on your face at 2 a.m.,
when I got home from my very first date.
I do not think that it's possible for anyone else to be as
    close
as you and I
We've been through it all, & thanks to Matilda,
I'll always be afraid to say bye.
I would feel sick & get all teary-eyed switching houses
between you and dad;
But you're such a great mom & he's such a great dad
that I always felt so sad.
I hope that I will never forget your worry-free, optimistic
    view;
I always felt better after a game of pool and quality talk-
    time with you.
Or your lifelong approach & philosophy of "people
    should always
come first" & knowing you had the willpower
& never drank, did drugs, or cursed.
As my mother you have given a special meaning
to 9 o'clock on Monday night;
Take off the phone, pop up some popcorn,
and watch "Raymond" in delight.
You can ALWAYS make me smile and laugh whether
you are trying or not;
Like the back-to-back Easters you hid my basket
in the same spot & forgot!
Your "motherly" traits, I must admit, at times are a bit out
    of place;
Like your Belgian waffle dinner that left us
starving & turned into a disgrace!
Or what is an "iron" and excuse me, but did I just hear you
    say "sew"?

But give you a ball, & and believe it or not,
you'll show me the right way to throw.
Our mother/son bond is so strong that there's no chance
that it will be beaten;
And, oh by the way, your strawberry jam,
is always some real good eatin'.
I still love it each night you come to my room,
say "good night" & tuck me in;
And as for the tennis, yes,
you are welcome for me always letting you win.
After 30 years of long and hard work,
you can kick back, relax, and retire;
You'll have time to come visit,
to make sure I don't set my dorm room on fire!
You've been such a great mom through my 18 years;
Thinking of leaving brings me oh so many tears.
So on this Mother's Day celebration;
there is just one thing I want you to hear;
That you're the best mom the world has to offer,
every single day of the year.
And if you ever feel as though you're stressed
or stuck in a dirty puddle;
Just know I will always be there for you,
and I'll never be too old to cuddle.
I love you mom
TJ Whammer

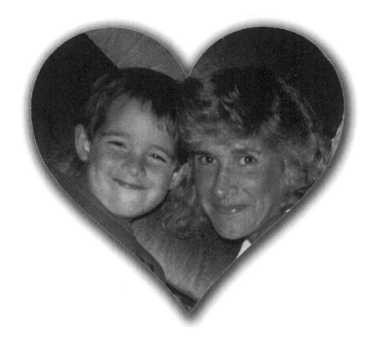

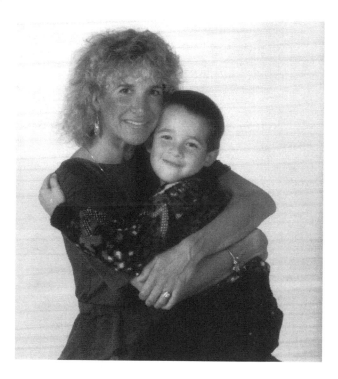

In their starvation state, anorexics seem to become someone else, unrecognizable, as if they are possessed. Many of them think of ED (Eating Disorder) as a person who becomes their friend. They hear ED's voice louder and stronger than any other.

TJ allowed me to take pictures of him when he was at a dangerously low weight so that maybe—just maybe—he could help someone else.

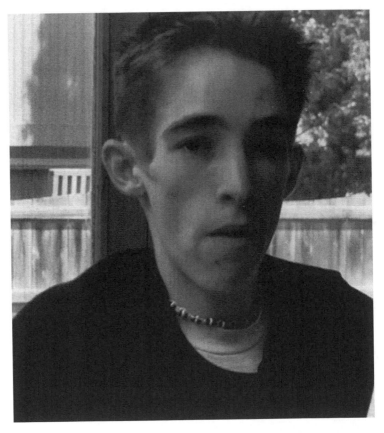

Before and after three months of residential treatment.

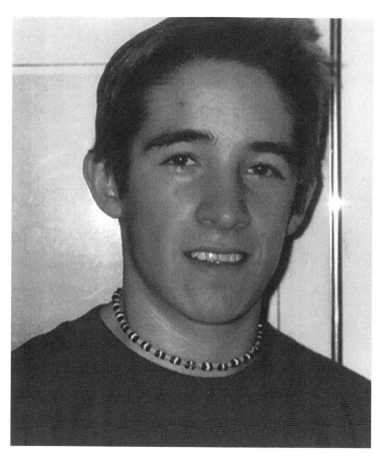

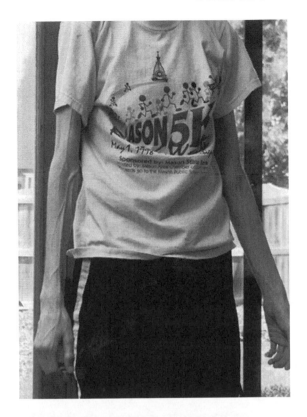

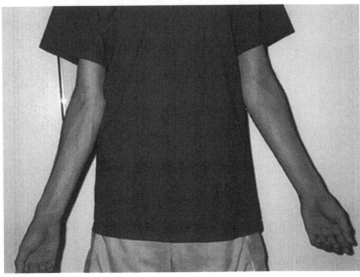

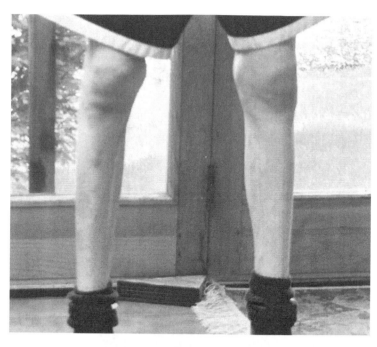

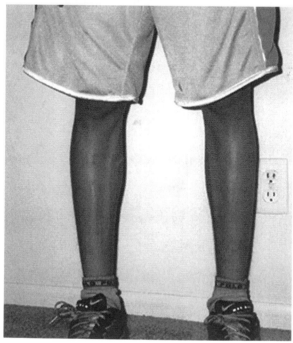

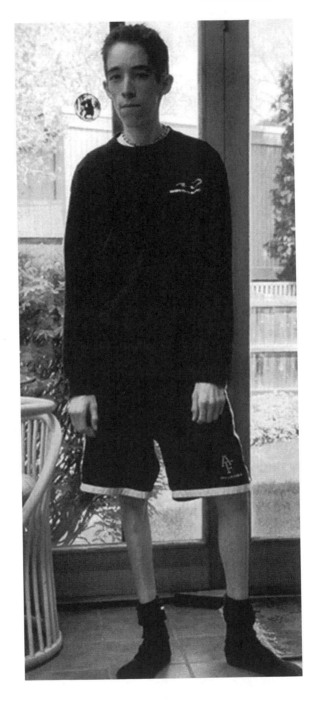

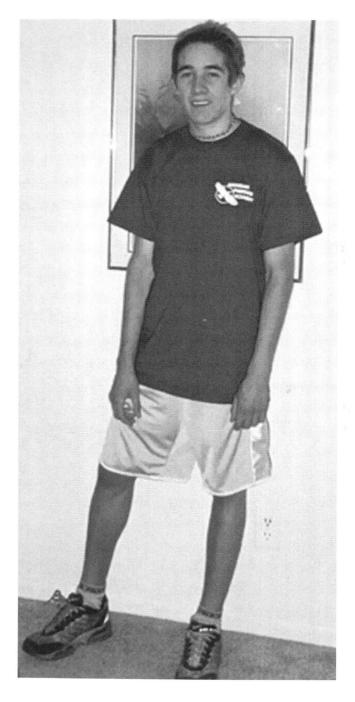

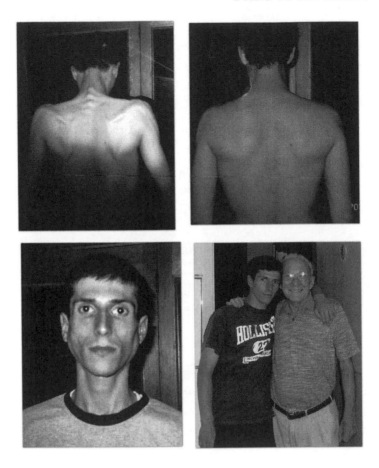

TJ's friend who sought residential treatment after TJ's passing.
Before and after 2007. Three months of residential treatment.

People ask why TJ wanted to commit a slow suicide. Is that
what people do with a terminal illness—want to die? TJ
wrote this in high school when he was first struggling with
anorexia. Do his words sound like someone wanting to die?

I am a very fortunate person who has been blessed with
a lot. There is so much that I have to be thankful for at
this point in my life. It's hard to choose one specific gift

or ability that I am most grateful for, but all of them com-
bined make me a pretty lucky person. I just hope that I
will never take anything for granted and always make the
most of my potential in life. It's scary to think of what my
life would be like without everything I have been blessed
with and am able to do.

If I had to choose, I would say that I am most grateful
for my mother and my father. They have taught me everything I know and provided me with so many valuable
lessons. My parents have always cared for me and done
what they thought best, and I am grateful for that. They
have provided food, a warm home, clothes, church, freedom, and kindness to me, something that not all children
can say. I am so glad that they had a Christian influence
on me as I grew up. Many children have no exposure to
Christian life but I have had the Lord in my life from a
very young age. I don't even want to think of what my
life would be like if that were not the case. My mom and
dad have provided me with so many experiences and
exposed me to so many opportunities that I can't possibly
be grateful enough. They have taught me almost every
sport, traveled with me across America, and given me
insight into what is right and wrong. I'm just grateful to
have parents like mine to help me get off to a good start
in life. Some kids find themselves at a disadvantage from
Day One because of their parents and the situation they
are in. [*The teacher inserted at the end of paragraph, "You
are amazing, TJ. I want a son like you someday."*]

Also, I am extremely grateful for my health. I can't even
imagine what I would do if I couldn't be active and carry
on everyday activities without my health. I think I would
go crazy. I am so thankful that I am able to play sports, be
healthy, and not have any physical disability restricting
me from doing so. I hear stories and know some people

that can't participate in the things they love most because of a handicap and I just thank God that I am healthy and able to do what I enjoy most. *[The teacher inserted at the end of the paragraph, "Wow. I am in awe of you TJ. You are a blessing."]*

I am thankful for my determination and willpower that God has given to me. I have a lot of dedication to succeed in life and accomplish what I set out for, and I'm just grateful that the Lord has blessed me with such a characteristic. Right now I notice people who shrug off their homework or don't go to practice because they just don't feel like it or don't care. I have enough determination, though, to convince myself to do what is right no matter how hard it is.

These high school writings are a bit more introspective, but I still see no evidence of anything self-destructive or very different from what many teenagers say and feel.

If I had the chance to live high school and my childhood all over again, there would be a few things that I would change. However, I would rather and more likely change the situations that I was in over how I responded to them. I think that given my situations, aspirations, and priorities of my life, right now I would not change too much in regard to how I lived my life.

I spend a lot of time doing schoolwork and studying to get good grades. My mom says that I study too much and should enjoy my childhood while I still can. But the way I see it is that I need to get good grades and study hard now so that I can get into a good college and in turn have a good and successful career when I get older. If I work hard now, it will surely pay off in the future. Plus, it's not like I don't have any fun now . . . I go out every weekend and do stuff with friends, I have a girlfriend, I play tennis, lift weights, run, ski, and do all the things I enjoy doing. I just spend a lot of time concentrating on school. If it were up to me, something I would change would be to have less homework and pressure to do well in high school. Basically I wouldn't change the fact that I worked so hard, but I wish the system and society wouldn't put so much pressure on high-school kids to grow up so fast.

I worked a *lot* this past summer for my dad, helping on the roofs, starting my own power-washing business, and cutting seven lawns per week. All summer, the only thing I heard from my mom was, "You're working too hard! Have some fun with your friends!" I did feel I worked too many hours and wish that I had spent more time with friends... but not that much because I made a *lot* of money over the summer. In turn, I was able to help pay ($5,000) for my brand new 2001 4X4 5–10 pickup, and even got to invest some in the stock market. So once again, it will "pay" off. I want to be well off in my future, so now is a good time to get the work habits down and start earning money.

I just wish my parents weren't divorced, because I would die to be able to sit down at the dinner table or watch a movie or open Christmas presents with both of them at the same time. But, that is nothing I can change or do over. IT IS BEYOND MY CONTROL. [*The caps are Susan's.*]

I underlined the parts of this next piece by TJ that clearly indicate his growing insecurity about becoming an adult and leaving his parents.

Most people are anxious and eager to get out of high school and go into college. I, on the other hand, am not. I think that most high-schoolers usually want to go to college for a number of reasons, including having conflicts with their parents. That was not an issue in my life. The party group desperately desires the freedom to go out and drink, smoke and misbehave away from the watchful eyes of their parents. I don't do any of that, so the freedom from my parents doesn't matter because they have trust in me. I already can basically do what I want or go where I want anyway because of their confidence in my decision-making.

Others might just not get along with their parents at all and can't wait to get away from the household. My relationship with my mom and dad is great, though. I would spend time with them just as quickly as with any of my friends. We have a lot in common and get along great. My mom and I play tennis, ski, run, and are active together. My dad and I go up north, ski, and hunt together. I really am going to miss not seeing them and spending time with them. Today I can come home from the school day and go play tennis with my mom or snowmobile with my dad. In six months, I will possibly be in another state and would have to fly halfway across the country to do something like that!

I also think that I will miss the schooling part of high school. From what I hear, college classes are loaded with people, the professors don't care about the kids and are very impersonal, and it's flat out hard! I like the high school set up where you have to go to class and you have to do your homework. In college, neither is required, and I prefer the more restrictive style. Also, I enjoy getting to know my teachers and having a friendly relationship with them. With so many kids in the classes, college professors probably won't even know my name! In high school, all the adults tell kids to have fun and

enjoy themselves now, because it is the best time of
our lives and it's all downhill from here! That's a little
scary seeing as how I only have five more months of that
left.

In high school I am still taken care of and have little
worries. My parents buy what I want for groceries, make
what I want for dinner, and serve all of my basic needs.
But I am on my own in college. Also the comparatively
small atmosphere of high school allows me to know everybody and be involved in everything. I'll be lucky to
have more than a handful of friends and to be active in
a couple of groups. What it basically comes down to is
that I don't really want to go to college . . . at all. I would
prefer not to have such a dramatic change, because I am
not ready to be an adult yet.

*Anorexics are often obsessive-compulsive. These expense lists
were found in TJ's lockbox and I was shocked when I saw
them. All of those returned Christmas presents! All of that
precision, control and self-sacrifice.*

DATE	INCOME	EXPENSE	DESCRIPTION
2/22/2003			
3/15/2003		6.50	"Old School" w/ Dan, Vick, & Dow
1/11/2003		8.50	Jimmy John's w/ Ashley
3/1/2003		15.00	"Lion King" w/ Ashley
3/5/2003	16.00		Meijer returns
3/5/2003	100.00		EDC check
1/11/2003	27.00		Eddie Bauer refund
3/5/2003	20.00		Aeropostale return
3/15/2003	5.00		Found in dorm

DATE	INCOME	EXPENSE	DESCRIPTION
3/19/2003		5.00	Serena CD
3/29/2003		5.00	NCAA tournament
3/30/2003	24.00		Returns
4/12/2003	5.00		MSU bet with Dad
4/18/2003		3.00	Blockbuster w/ Ashley
4/18/2003	10.00		Barb's birthday gift
1/1/2003	205.00		Birthday money
6/11/2003	10.00		Bookstore return
6/15/2003	30.00		Hawkins graduation gift
6/15/2003	7.00		Returns
6/28/2003		7.00	Father's Day
6/28/2003		1412.13	Car repair
6/28/2003		32.00	Phone bill
7/4/2003		80.00	Speeding ticket
7/5/2003		5.50	"Terminator 3" w/ Nick & Andy
7/9/2003	9.25		Golf refund from Indian Hills
7/27/2003		6.50	Movie, "Matrix Reloaded" w/Dad
8/5/2003		5.00	Movie w/Ashley
8/7/2003		2.00	Bowling with Jessie
8/12/2003		5.00	Movie, ice cream w/ Ashley & Vamsi
8/12/2003	105.00		Watch return refund
8/19/2003		5.00	Driver's license renewal
8/19/2003	4766.29		1st work check (before expenses)
8/21/2003	3939.00		2nd work check
8/11/2003	1087.00		3rd work check

DATE	INCOME	EXPENSE	DESCRIPTION
8/24/2003	340.00		Painting for Rich
8/24/2003	225.00		Vi's lawn (all summer)
8/24/2003	350.00		New lawn (all summer)
8/23/2003	10.00		Leftover cash
8/23/2003	75.00		Sold Chemistry & Statistics
8/24/2003		70.00	Books
6/1/2003	75.00		Sold Calculus book
6/22/2003	55.00		Sold Economic book
8/29/2003	8.00		Trim and weed for Vi
8/31/2003	9.50		Weed for Vi
8/30/2003		10.00	TUPAC/Snoop poster
8/31/2003	55.00		Vi lawn
9/6/2003	9.50		MSU ticket sales
9/6/2003	15.00		Leftover cash
9/13/2003	25.00		Vi lawn
9/14/2003	10.00		New lawn
9/20/2003	25.00		Vi lawn
9/20/2003	15.00		New lawn
9/27/2003	25.00		Vi lawn
9/27/2003	15.00		New lawn
10/4/2003	25.00		Vi lawn
10/4/2003	15.00		New lawn
10/17/2003	25.00		Vi lawn
10/17/2003	15.00		New lawn
11/27/2003	25.00		Vi lawn
12/22/2003	5.00		New lawn
12/22/2003	17.38		Poker at Thanksgiving

DATE	INCOME	EXPENSE	DESCRIPTION
12/22/2003	120.00		Christmas presents
12/25/2003	2.59		Christmas money
12/24/2003	50.00		Returns
12/29/2003	2.00		Christmas money
12/29/2003	100.00		Extra
12/29/2003		1317.84	Driving classes
12/29/2003	12.74		Work check
12/25/2003	11.35		Christmas money
12/25/2003	150.00		Ashley Christmas present
		100.00	Christmas present (phone)

Total Income	$13,628.21		
Total Expense		$1,756.36	
Net Income	$11,871.85		

This shopping receipt was also found 11/26/05:

Mega warmer	$1.19
Mega warmer	1.19
Toe warmer	1.49
Toe warmer	1.49
Body warmer	1.49
Body warmer	1.49
Jump rope	2.99
Body warmer	3.99
Gum	.99
Chicken broth	.99
Fat-free butter spray	1.59
Fat-free butter spray	1.59
Fat-free butter spray	1.59
Fat-free butter spray	1.59

Gum	1.79
Gum	1.99
Gum	1.99
Gum	1.99
Gum	1.99
Gum	1.99
Seasoning	1.99
Seasoning	1.99
Gum	2.09
Gum	2.09
Fat-free Pringles	2.09
Fat-free Pringles	2.09
Gum	2.29
Fat-free cottage cheese	2.39
Seasoning	2.59
Seasoning	2.59
Jell-O	2.50
Jell-O	2.50
Fat-free syrup	2.50
Fat-free syrup	2.50
Fat-free syrup	2.50
Fat-free syrup	2.50
Fat-free syrup	2.50
Cereal	3/7.00
Cereal	3/7.00
Cereal	3/7.00

Three years after TJ's passing, his best friend Daniel was reading a book called Confessions of a Scholarship Judge: How to Win More Money by Learning What Judges Hate! *by Josh Barsch. In it, a scholarship judge gives good and solid advice on how to write an essay to earn scholarship money. He chose 19 essays to give as examples of excellent writing. The author put his comments in bold print in order to emphasize what constitutes an exceptional essay.*

Imagine Daniel reading this book in his living room, oblivious to the fact that the next page he turned would have "TJ Warschefsky" at the top! He told me he nearly passed out. I almost did the same when I read the author's comments . . . especially his final one.

TJ WARSCHEFSKY

3,2,1 . . . Liftoff! The earth shook, the sky illuminated, and everybody stood in awe. My Uncle Jerry had just blasted into outer space for a five-month stay aboard the space station MIR. Noticing the tears running down everyone's face, it was right then that I told myself I, too, would accomplish something significant one day. I wanted to have an impact on people, and I wanted to make a difference. I would learn in the following years that making a difference comes in many forms and finding my niche would be my challenge. [**Nice intro . . . it's unique that he was actually present as his uncle was blasted into space, and I can see how the reaction of the crowd might be one of those moments that inspired you to do great things of your own. I'm intrigued . . .**]

In my Uncle's book, he wrote: "Specialization is for insects. Man should be able to change a diaper, run a marathon, build a house, write a book, appreciate good music, and fly in space." I value a balanced lifestyle and think it is important to be well rounded in order to interact with people of varying backgrounds and beliefs. [**A mature thought from a young adult. Nice to hear.**] I knew I would someday have to modify the last part of my uncle's quote about flying in space, and replace it with whatever I found my passion to be.

I always wanted a career where I would wake up every morning and be excited to go to work. [**Don't we all!**] Perhaps that is why it took me such a long time to decide on a career. There were many tasks that I was skilled in, and there were aspects of certain jobs that I enjoyed, but I always knew there was that perfect niche waiting for me. There are three principle responsibilities that I desire for my profession; I want to be a businessman. I want to be a doctor. I want to be a community leader and family man.

I began a lawn business when I was in seventh grade, and business has always come naturally to me. My entrepreneurial spirit and talent in business drew me to Albion College, where I would study liberal arts and major in business. At Albion College, I planned to compete on the tennis and cross-country teams, and I received scholarships in both the Gerstacker Honors Institute for Professional Management and the Ford Institute for Public Policy and Service. The public policy program appealed to me because it allowed me to continue my community service. I got involved in many campus organizations, including being Treasurer of the Investment Club, the Vice President of Albion College Pre-dental Club, and a member of the National Service Fraternity, Alpha Psi Omega. [**Note: This is a service fraternity and therefore isn't what I refer to in the section on Greek life.**]

During my very first semester, I left campus to help out with an urgent illness in my family. My professors allowed me to complete my courses, although some professors chose to give me "credit" instead of a letter grade, but I was willing to accept that consequence to help my family. I returned that spring with more direction and a change of heart. I knew I wanted to be in health-care, because

I wanted to help others. I realize that is a stereotypical response, however, it strikes a much more personal note for me. My stepfather suffers from multiple sclerosis, and I have taken on the responsibility of "man of the house" and "caregiver" for as long as I can remember. [**YES! Remember what I said about telling the committee about your responsibilities within your own family? This is a perfect example.**] Helping him and my family always gave me so much satisfaction. As a doctor, a dentist is prepared to work with their hands everyday and yield noticeable results while at the same time diagnosing a multitude of other health-related measures. I knew that I had to find something that allowed me to interact and help people, and my extensive business skills and creativity could be utilized in running my own office. I was determined to complete my studies in business and public policy, but I also began courses for a pre-health career path. [**A mature choice, blending science with business. If he follows through, TJ will be very well off someday.**]

Organization, time management, discipline, and an exceptional memory had always been strong aspects of my character. [**Ditto, then, what I just said about probably making it big someday.**] However, my intense course load (including online and summer courses), community service (both at home and at college), varsity sports, work, and extracurricular involvement were an obvious over-commitment. I was able to manage my numerous obligations and activities, but realized that I needed to narrow my pursuits in order to be most effective and efficient. I gained valuable insight from this period of over-commitment, as it taught me how to handle the boundaries of my limits and the importance of a balanced lifestyle. [**Mature observation. In most** cases, students recount this load of activities with a trite phrase like "I stay busy managing my friends, work, classes, etc.," but TJ gleans a lesson that too much is too much. As you can tell, TJ is painting a picture of himself as a pretty mature guy, which is the advice I give in "Confessions".]

An internship experience with a CPA and financial planning firm verified that I would not enjoy a desk job. I needed to be on my feet and interacting with people. I sought out the career development office and took career interest and personal inventories. My love for volunteerism, outstanding eye-hand coordination, interest in art and piano, work ethic, people skills, drive and motivation for success, knack for business, and my leadership traits—all combine to reveal that dentistry was the profession for me. [**Wow, I'd have never put that together. But come to think of it, I guess that stuff would all make you a good dentist.**] I felt as though I could have a more significant and successful impact on the lives of others if I translated those business skills and applied them to a greater cause. As a dentist, business skills are particularly important, as each patient I will treat is essentially a client; but at the same time, I am able to further their health and well-being.

I contacted every dentist I knew and began to observe at every opportunity. I even found a dental office where I could observe on a Saturday. I shadowed oral surgeons, endodontists, implant specialists, and orthodontists. From my very first observation, I knew that I was going to be a dentist. I loved interacting with patients and was interested in the concerns and strategies for oral health care and disease prevention. My love of school and learning is a perfect match, and I truly could not wait to begin my studies and career as a dentist.

It is becoming increasingly apparent that dentists are often the very first health care practitioners to recognize and diagnose medical problems. These ailments include diabetes, obesity, cardiovascular disease, cancer, eating disorders, and ADHD, among many others. [**Fascinating. I had no idea this was the case. And if a judge is, at any point, fascinated by your essay, that's a good thing.**] After just one semester in dental school, I have been amazed at the significant impact a dentist can have on the overall health and well-being of their patients. Dentists are not typically thought of as "doctors" in the wider health spectrum of the word, although numerous lives are saved each and every day because of a head, neck, and oral cavity examination performed by dentists and their resulting referrals.

In addition to recognition and diagnosis of several illnesses, the more specific oral-health care that dentists provide to their patients have a significant impact on their overall quality of life. Research has shown that oral health influences emotional, as well as physical, characteristics of everyday lives.

Individuals with poor oral health often miss work or school due to pain. Also, the increasing emphasis on cosmetic dentistry proves that it frequently results in a lack of self-confidence and embarrassment. Studies on children have revealed that one of the most common types of criticism they receive is related to their teeth, which can have a considerable impact on their emotional development. [**He's right. I'm a lot older than TJ, and I remember kids getting teased because of their teeth all the time.**]

With the baby boomer population advancing into the category of senior citizenship, the focus on this age group is becoming much more relevant. Lack of self-confidence and poor nutrition are two of the major categories that result in the poor health of the elderly. Technology in dentistry has made it possible to treat patients of all ages and conditions, and can surely assist the elderly in their quality of life.

As a dentist, I am undertaking one of the most diversified occupations in terms of the responsibilities I have and the impact that can result. I am immensely intrigued with the opportunity to not only help the population have healthier and stronger teeth, but to also recognize other life-threatening diseases, help with the emotional security that comes with cosmetics, and relieve the stresses and pains that can so profoundly arise from poor oral health. My uncle lived up to the cliché of reaching for the stars. [**Way to come full circle!**] While I may not be flying among the stars, I have found the perfect goal for me. To modify his quote:

> Specialization is for insects. Man should be able to change a diaper, run a marathon, build a house, write a book, appreciate good music, and fill a cavity.

[A mature and interesting essay from a kid who has tons of promise, and those are the kinds of kids we like to give scholarships to. Very well done.]

18

"My God, Now What Do I Do?": Advice for Parents

STEP ONE: ADMIT AND FACE

At this point, you may be thinking, "My child does not exhibit all or even most of the behaviors or symptoms described." Please understand: It truly does not matter what he weighs. *He can be in danger at any weight.* Often, bulimics look "normal."

Any person struggling with an eating disorder is using food and weight to deal with his emotions. One of the biggest challenges parents face is the very same thing their child is facing: *admitting there is a problem.*

People with eating disorders do everything in their power to hide it. Ordinarily honest people become skilled liars who will say anything to protect their illness. The disease is their friend, their security, their comfort, their control, their accomplishment, their everything. They will tell you nothing is wrong, that they are training for this or that or just trying to lose a couple of pounds, no big deal. Like addicts of all kinds, they believe they can stop whenever they choose. And it may, in fact, start out that way. I truly feel that there is a specific point in the course of the illness when a switch is flipped and an anorexic's behavior becomes totally out of his control. He finds himself in a downward spiral and can't change the course of it.

Parents and loved ones have as hard a time admitting that the disease has come into their lives as their children do. And even after they've admitted it to themselves, it is very difficult for them to share the fact with others. From my own experiences, I know that one reason for this is feelings of guilt—the concern that others will think it's their fault.

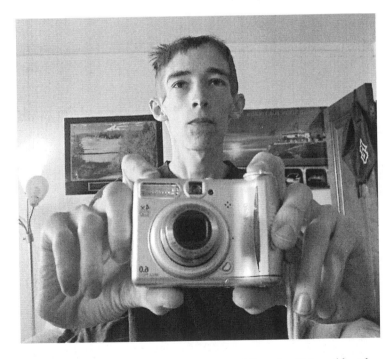

We found several disturbing pictures TJ took of himself with the digital camera he got for his last Christmas . . . most too horrific to share. I include this one because it shows his once beautiful, sparkling eyes looking vacant and possessed. This is not TJ—not a person I recognize.

Over the eight-and-a-half years of TJ's struggle, I had to answer many questions and listen to a lot of well-meaning advice from people who had no idea what his illness was about. They said things like:

- "It's just a phase. He'll snap out of it."
- "Just make TJ sit at the table until he finishes his plate of food!"
- "Leave him alone. He'll eat when he's hungry."
- "I don't care if he eats bird seed as long as he eats some thing!"
- "Well, Susan, cooking was never one of your strong points. Why don't you have TJ come live with us for the summer?"
- "Let me talk to TJ from a medical point of view, and I can tell him what these test numbers mean."
- "Let me talk to TJ from a spiritual point of view, and I can tell him that the Bible says to treat your body like a temple."
- "Let me talk to TJ from an athletic point of view because he isn't able to perform in sports using his God-given talent."
- "Why does he want to kill himself?"

STEP TWO: ACT YESTERDAY

This was not the step I struggled with. I acted immediately. When I saw TJ without his shirt at that high school soccer party, I immediately made an appointment with the pediatrician. In TJ's case, early (and relentless) action didn't save the day—but I cannot stress enough the urgency of this step. It is *vitally* important that you act immediately. Notice that I didn't say "after he graduates" or "after the upcoming wedding" or "right after our summer trip." With each passing week, the illness becomes worse. Just as with cancer, if you catch and treat it early, there is a much better chance of success. The longer the wait, the worse the odds.

Remember, also, that the situation gets much more complicated once your child turns 18. At that point, you will have no access to his medical records. Authorities won't even tell you what he weighs. The issue of privacy rights becomes horrendous—and I'll say it again: I believe that eating disorders should be considered an exception to the rules because with this illness, *the patient does not want to get well!*

I believe the most common mistake parents make is trying to keep everything in their child's life as normal as possible—which means squeezing in a therapist appointment after school and basketball practice. We want our children to fit in: to finish high school with their class, start college with their friends, finish their sports season, etc. But absolutely none of that matters if they are ill. All of TJ's honors, scholarships, good grades, awards, acceptance letters, trophies, and even bank accounts didn't matter in the end. Your child can start, finish, accomplish . . . later. Nothing else really matters if he doesn't have his health or his life.

As frantic parents facing a condition we don't understand, the first thing we are likely to do is search for information anywhere we can find it. We spend hours looking at books in the library and at bookstores, peruse the Internet, and end up overwhelmed and in a state of panic.

Most of the books I found when I started to research

TJ's problem concentrated on what type of person might be predisposed to this illness. The list included perfectionists, overachievers, and people pleasers. (Bingo.) From the outside, they appear to have it "all together," but inside they feel helpless, inadequate, worthless, and never good enough. (Very interesting.) They have high levels of Cortisol (brain hormones most related to stress) and decreased levels of Serotonin and Norepinephrine, which are associated with feelings of well-being. (So it *is* a medical condition after all!)

The books also helped me identify the signs that my child was struggling with an eating disorder, and that was very helpful. What they didn't tell me was what to do right away; what number to call today!

In my search for professionals to help TJ, I discovered that many therapists are not trained to treat eating disorders. You need to find a person or team specifically trained in treating anorexia and bulimia. Don't be afraid to ask questions like, "How many clients have you worked with who have eating disorders? How many of those clients are doing well now?" If you are fortunate enough to find an expert in this area, you should see improvement—but never stop monitoring the situation.

Sad to say, you can't trust your anorexic child on the subject of food, exercise or weight. "I ate a big meal earlier," shouldn't convince you of anything. The only real proof is the number on the scale. And even weigh-ins can be deceiving. You've read about how TJ manipulated the numbers and there are plenty of other tricks, too, from drinking lots of fluids before the weigh-in to hiding weights in the bottom of socks, or in pockets and hoods.

If I had to do it over again, I would have put TJ in a residential treatment center immediately and skipped the therapists and dieticians. Why? For example, TJ said he would gain weight if he could put on solid muscle and no fat, so we hired him a personal trainer for a month. The trainer was extremely impressed with TJ because he had memorized the calories and fat content of everything she told him to eat, as well as all of the exercises she gave him. What did he do when he got home? Ate his usual diet and *added* the new exercises to his already insane exercise routine.

Until an anorexic achieves a healthy weight, he can't be reached by therapy because his mind isn't functioning normally. It's that simple. He could have the best therapy session possible, but won't come home and make a sandwich. Residential stays are designed to enforce new behaviors and bring the mind to a point where therapy can actually work. Most anorexics enjoy watching others eat and will go out of their way to make or serve food without touching any themselves. They do *not* enjoy seeing others exercise, though, especially if they are not exercising themselves at that moment. *Their sense of discipline and control are diminished when they witness discipline and control in others.* Again, early intervention can help stop this downward slide—and the process of becoming a "better and better" anorexic.

Again, I wish I had skipped all of the less effective steps and not worried about what TJ would be missing during a three-month stay at a residential center. With every week that passed, the illness became more ingrained.

How do you find the right residential treatment center? This is where the Internet does help. Once you find some possibilities, you need to find out which of them your insurance will cover. If you have a son who needs help the situation is a little harder, as there currently are not very many centers that accommodate males. But (sadly), with the rising incidence of male eating disorders, this is likely to improve. (By 2012, the rate of males suffering from eating disorders had risen dramatically to one in four.)

The key is getting your child somewhere as soon as possible and ensuring that he stays as long as he needs to, often three to six months. Next, you must hope that your insurance will cover most of the cost. Residential treatment is very expensive, ranging from $500 to $2000 a day—an average of $30,000 a month. Without help from our insurance companies, most of us couldn't manage the cost.

As I described in telling TJ's story, it is the patient who must "make the call" to get into treatment, and if he is over 18, he must submit to the interview on his own. He has to say that he wants to be there. This can create great tension in the family, because most anorexics do *not* want to go!

When I was grappling with this situation, I got very angry. It seemed to me that the experts should understand that TJ wasn't interested in acting in his own best interest. But I also understood—and you should, too—that if a patient is not committed to getting well, he won't make progress. As TJ's friend Daniel described, he can just do and say whatever he needs to in order to get out and resume his old patterns.

There is a powerless feeling associated with this step. We told TJ we would not pay for college if he didn't go to treatment first; that we would take away his car, his insurance, whatever we could think of to bribe him to make the call. And I'm glad we finally prevailed. My advice is that you should do anything you can think of to force your child to make that call. Leave the issue of his ongoing commitment to getting better to the experts once he is admitted.

Once he is in treatment, you must do all you can to keep him there as long as possible. That means closing your ears to his crying and pleas. Let the experts decide when release is appropriate. I can still hear my son bargaining and trying to pull at my heartstrings: "I get this, Mom," he said over and over. "Please let me start back to college [or come home for Christmas, or whatever]. I don't want to miss a whole semester because they want me here for two more weeks! I'll see a therapist and a dietician and a medical doctor as often as you want. I'll sign a contract! Let me go back to college and eat their good food instead of this nasty stuff. I've been compliant, Mom. I want to stay well! Please trust and believe in me, Mom. Please."

I know how hard it is to resist your child's pleas, but I urge you to be strong.

Because our family was fractured by divorce and re-marriage, it was hard for us to present a united front—but this is extremely important in combating your child's attempts to manipulate and control you. If he can, he'll pit you against one another. Get together, talk things through, and agree to agree. Stay the course. Remember, you all share a deep love for your child, and that is a good basis for sticking together on his treatment.

Say to yourself, "I am the meanest mom in the world, but that's OK! I'm saving my kid's life. I can accept being hated now in return for being loved later."

Even if you do everything right, a relapse is very likely. If cancer comes back, you don't hesitate to return for more treatment. Same idea. You've read the story of TJ's best friend, Daniel, who went back to residential *four* times before he found the strength to heal and pursue his happy ending.

Don't be discouraged if residential treatment doesn't work the first time. If your child is doing well six months after his residential stay, his chances of success are very good. Here's a recap of TJ's treatments—eloquent evidence of the tenacity of this disease and the importance of staying the course.

TJ's Residential Treatments

First stay
Admission: 10/25/02
Discharge (Against Medical Advice): 1/9/03
Weight gained: 19.2 lbs

Second stay
Admission: 5/10/05
Discharge: 8/14/05
Weight gained: 37 lbs

Third stay
Admission: 7/11/06
Discharge (Against Medical Advice): 8/11/06
Weight gained: 4.6 lbs

STEP THREE: RETURNING HOME

This can be the most important step in the successful treatment of eating disorders, but for me, it was the most difficult. What should we as family members do upon the return of our loved one from treatment? The experts provide very little guidance—perhaps because they don't know all the answers either.

TJ was discharged with a packet of information, but it

did little to ease my deep fear and concern. The first time he skipped lunch, the first time he drove off to the club to work out, the first time he reached for fat-free cereal, I didn't know how to react. I was told not to become the "food police"—but what exactly does that mean? Was I supposed to back off entirely and let TJ return to his old, destructive behaviors without a fight?

"Aren't you going to have lunch, honey?"

"Don't worry about it, Mom. You're not supposed to do that."

Then what?

I was told to throw away the scale in the house but it was a snap for TJ to find another one. I was told to get rid of his small-sized clothes, but most of them had been hanging on him and now fit a little better.

The most crucial advice I can offer you (based on my personal downfall in our journey), is, be careful about letting your child leave home. I should not have let TJ go back to school. I should not have let him resume living alone. I should not have let him return to the stress and isolation of that environment. I wish I could have protected and supported him more during that very scary transition period from Rogers Residential to our house and then quickly back to college. It was too easy for him to revert to old behaviors when faced with familiar stressors and triggers. At residential, he had been cared for and protected. He had made friends who understood and shared his situation. He was not isolated or embarrassed. Back in the real world, his old friend the eating disorder was waiting with open arms.

I've thought a lot about what might ease this difficult transition for others, and I wonder if maybe anorexics need some sort of halfway house. Once they've spent the time necessary in a residential treatment center, perhaps they could be discharged to a group home where they could plan, shop for, and cook their own meals. It might be a place where they'd spend only part of their time, sharing their thoughts and fears in group therapy sessions and gradually working their way back into the real world. Depending on how well they maintained their weight and good attitude, their stay could be longer or shorter—and if they really started losing ground, they could be sent back to residential.

Throwing these fragile individuals right back into the real world doesn't seem to succeed, especially for males. Perhaps boys find it more difficult to relinquish control, or are more resistant to therapy than girls. Clearly, their bodies send them different signals. (Females stop menstruating, for example—scary and concrete evidence that they are damaging their bodies—while a lowered testosterone level in boys isn't tangible to them.)

Until the medical establishment recognizes that a gradual transition back to independence is crucial, families are left trying to create a safe, controlled environment that is conducive to continuing recovery. If your child comes home and starts losing weight, he needs to return to treatment. If he maintains a healthy weight for a significant amount of time, his privileges can be carefully expanded.

An eating disorder is hard to understand, hard to fix, and very frustrating. Anorexics and bulimics need love and support and gentle discussions, but they also need a watchful eye and consistency. And parents of these children have needs, too. Most important, we need other adults to talk to who understand our situation. It is entirely too difficult to go through this process alone. Support from spouses, family members, friends, and possibly a counselor or therapist is crucial. After all, we can't help our children unless we are emotionally steady ourselves.

A united family is vital. Support groups for families dealing with eating disorders are badly needed! The college community in which we live in has support groups for everything: divorce, separation, widowhood, overeating, alcoholism, single parenthood, illness, abuse, grief, disability, nicotine, Alzheimer's, Parkinson's, OCD, job loss, schizophrenia, postpartum depression . . . but *nothing* for families dealing with eating disorders!

There is still a lot of work to be done in tackling an illness that affects 11 million Americans. According to the National Eating Disorder Association, between 2000 and 2006, eating disorder hospitalizations for children under 12 more than doubled. The constant barrage of unrealistic body images that bombards our kids via all forms of media is forcing them to focus on how they look rather than who they are. That is unlikely to change. We can only try to be aware of the damage this can do, be vigilant for signs of disordered thinking and behavior in our children, and try to instill in them a sense that there are more important things in life than how we look and how much we weigh.

Why did I let TJ go back to dental school? Why did the hospital let him out after that final stay, when he was obviously so terribly ill? Why couldn't someone have fixed him? Why, with all of his intelligence and drive couldn't he *just eat*?

TJ had everything going for him. He could not have been more loved. I'll never understand his journey into anorexia, just as I still can't believe he's really gone. But if this book can help save lives, it can help me make some sense of it all. I have comforted myself with the thought that perhaps God allows suffering in order to breed in us a passion for reaching out and helping others.

Until I see my son again, I will breathe in and breathe out believing that he left a great legacy. He made a difference and inspired me to try to do the same. I miss him every single minute of every single day. But, I think he is proud of me for writing this book and telling his story. What more can a mother ask for?

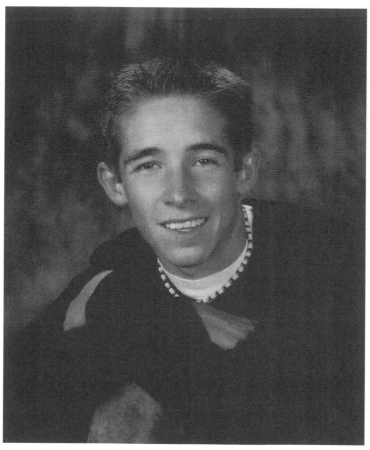

Thomas Lee "TJ" Warschefsky II
April 18, 1984—February 14, 2007

ABOUT THE AUTHOR

SUSAN BARRY graduated from Michigan State University with a Masters degree and taught elementary school for thirty years, until her retirement. She is an avid tennis player and has twice played in national championships. After her son's passing, she started a support group, has helped more than thirty families around the country navigate the struggle against eating disorders, given talks at several universities, held five charity races in TJ's memory, and raised thousands of dollars for research into cures. She lives in Michigan with her husband John and daughter Jessica.

To learn more about her fund-raising efforts and make a contribution to TJ's Fund for Eating Disorder Research, go to aedweb.org and click on "Get Involved," "Donate," and "TJ's Fund."

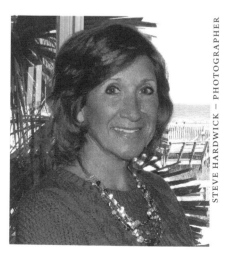

STEVE HARDWICK – PHOTOGRAPHER